AF364232

Bioequivalence Study of Drugs:

Its Facilities and Techniques

Bioequivalence Study of Drugs:

Its Facilities and Techniques

Bhaswati Pal

Shubhasis Dan

Tapan Kumar Pal

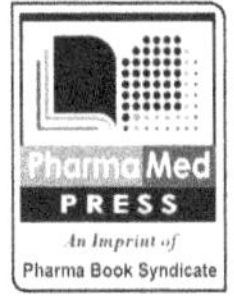

PharmaMed Press

An imprint of Pharma Book Syndicate

A unit of BSP Books Pvt. Ltd.

4-4-309/316, Giriraj Lane,

Sultan Bazar, Hyderabad - 500 095.

Bioequivalence Study of Drugs: Its Facilities and Techniques
by *Bhaswati Pal, Shubhasis Dan, and Tapan Kumar Pal*

© 2021, *by Publisher,* All rights reserved.

No part of this book or parts thereof may be reproduced, stored in a retrieval system or transmitted in any language or by any means, electronic, mechanical, photocopying, recording or otherwise without the prior written permission of the publishers.

Published by

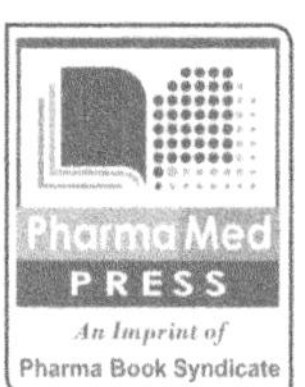

PharmaMed Press

An imprint of Pharma Book Syndicate

A unit of BSP Books Pvt. Ltd.

4-4-309/316, Giriraj Lane, Sultan Bazar, Hyderabad - 500 095.
Phone: 040-23445688, 23445600; Fax: 91+40-23445611
e-mail: info@pharmamedpress.com
www.pharmamedpress.com/pharmamedpress.net

ISBN: 978-93-88305-90-7

PREFACE

India is the largest provider of generic drugs globally with the Indian generics accounting for 20% of global exports in terms of volume. Comparative pharmacokinetic data under the regulatory framework of bioavailability and bioequivalence (BA/BE) study data is widely accepted by the developed countries regulatory agencies over last 4 decades to establish the efficacy of the generic products. With1.2 billion people and wide variety of diseases and patient pool makes this country very attractive to the pharmaceutical companies for conducting clinical research (Clinical trials, BA/BE studies). Besides large and diverse patient pool, we also have a large pool of pharmacist, scientists and engineers who are potential enough to steer the pharmaceutical industry to a higher level. India is the largest provider of generic drugs globally with the Indian generics accounting for 20% of global exports in terms of volume.

Availability of the generic products in the market has been gained serious public consideration in respect of their safety and efficacy with the innovator products. Bioequivalence (BE) studies with a view to demonstrate therapeutic equivalence between two drug products (test and reference or innovator) can able to answer this public concern internationally.

The concept of BA/BE study was developed and accepted by the developed countries regulatory agencies over last 4 decades. In the early 1970's, the "United States Food and Drug Administration" (US-FDA) became interested in biological availability of new drugs. They formed a committee to establish the pharmaceutical and therapeutic equivalence relationships of drugs which later on implemented as the Code of Federal Regulations (CFR) for the regulations of bioavailability.

Pharmacokinetics is the application of mathematical calculation and modeling techniques to the time course of absorption, distribution, metabolism, and excretion of drugs in the body. It is primarily concerned with the analysis of concentration and rate of drug availability to the required receptor site. Analysis of plasma samples will target concentration of drug as time progresses, resulting in the production of a 'plasma drug concentration-time curve'. Plasma drug concentration time curve can be obtained after a single oral dose of a drug by measuring concentration of drug in plasma samples taken at various intervals of time and plotting the concentration of drug in plasma vs corresponding time at which plasma samples were collected.

BE study can be coined as the comparative pharmacokinetic study, where the bioequivalence was established based on the following parameters of test and innovator drug product--maximum plasma concentration (Cmax), time to reach the maximum plasma concentration (Tmax), half-life ($t_{1/2}$): time taken for the plasma concentration to fall by 50% and area under the plasma concentration curve (AUC): a calculation to assess the bodies total exposure to a drug over a given time.

As on date (December, 2018), CDSCO approved only 82 bioequivalence study center in India. In India, as per Central Drug Standard Control Organization (CDSCO, Ministry of Health and Family Welfare, Government of India) requirements, there are two types of permission or approval required:

(A) Facility Specific Approval: A CRO can't undertake BA/BE Study unless it is accredited by the CDSCO.

(B) Study Specific Approval: CDSCO issues study protocol specific NOC for conducting that particular BA/BE Study.

As the aspect of bioequivalence study is not included in the syllabus of pharmacy or MBBS, this thesis will be definitely helpful to the pharmacist, doctors and the pharma industries to have a thorough knowledge regarding this subject as well as it will guide them to establish a Contract Research Organizations (CRO) for conducting BA/BE study. Moreover it is obvious that the technology transfer from existing CROs for conducting BA/BE study is not possible due to commercial reason. This book will definitely beneficial to them who are interested to proceed further in this field. This investigation covers the essential components required for a BA/BE center. To conduct a bioequivalence study of drugs the basic infrastructural facilities have been explained covering the following areas:

(a) Space;
(b) Instrumental Facilities;
(c) Manpower requirement.

The specimen layout plan for CPU (Clinical Pharmacological Unit) and the bioanalytical labs including the list of essential instruments for analyzing drug in plasma as per regulatory requirements has been attached. The list of SOPs (Standard Operating Procedure) for conducting BA/BE studies have been furnished for necessary guidance. Prior to any bioequivalence study the approval of ethics committee is mandatory. The procedure of getting the approval along with the composition of Ethics committee has been highlighted. The contents of protocol to conduct BA/BE study including ICF (Informed Consent Form), CRF (Case Record/Report Form), PIS (Patient Information Sheet), Investigator's Undertaking and preclinical study of volunteers have been discussed in details. The procedure for reporting SAE (Serious Adverse Event) is also a vital component of the protocol.

We shall be happy if the Pharmacists, Scientists and Researchers as well as Executives of the pharmaceutical industries are benefitted by going through this book. We would like to convey our sincere gratitude to our associated Clinical Pharmacologists, Prof. (Dr.) Sudeb Mondal, MD, Dr. Balaram Ghosh, MD, DM and Dr. Arunava Biswas, MD, DM for their kind and cordial support.

Lastly, the wholehearted support and technical help of Mrs. Alpana Pal, Managing Partner and the staffs of TAAB Biostudy Services, Kolkata inspired us to write this book. We are grateful to Mrs. A Pal.

Dr. Bhaswati Pal, MBA (Clinical)

Dr. Shubhasis Dan, M. Pharm, Ph. D
Prof. (Dr.) Tapan Kumar Pal, M. ChE (Gold Medalist),
Former DAAD Fellow (Germany) F.I.E, VDI (Germany)

CONTENTS

Preface .... (v)

Chapter 1

    Introduction 1

Chapter 2

    Essential Components required for BA/BE Study Centre 7

Chapter 3

    Ethical Perspectives 23

Chapter 4

    Pre-requisites for Conducting BA/BE Studies 31

Chapter 5

    Methods to Conduct BE Study 37

Chapter 6

    Contents of a BE Study Report 121

Chapter 7

    Summary 165

Chapter 8

    LC-MS/MS Instrumentation 183

Chapter 9

    References & Appendices 189

About the Authors 227

Chapter 1

Introduction

India adores a very significant position in the global pharmaceuticals market. With 1.2 billion people and wide variety of diseases and patient pool makes this country very attractive to the pharmaceutical companies for conducting clinical research (Clinical trials, BA/BE studies). Besides large and diverse patient pool, we also have a large pool of pharmacist, scientists and engineers who have potential to steer the pharmaceutical industry to a higher level. India is the largest provider of generic drugs globally with the Indian generics accounting for 20% of global exports in terms of volume [1].

Conceptual Idea of Bioequivalence Studies

Availability of the generic products in the market has gained serious public consideration with respect of their safety and efficacy with the innovator products. Bioequivalence (BE) studies with a view to demonstrate therapeutic equivalence between two drug products (test and reference or innovator) can be able to answer this public concern internationally.

The concept of BA/BE study was developed and accepted by the developed countries regulatory agencies over last 4 decades. In the early 1970's, the "United States Food and Drug Administration" (US-FDA) became interested in biological availability of new drugs. They formed a committee to establish the pharmaceutical and therapeutic equivalence relationships of drugs which later on implemented as the Code of Federal Regulations (CFR) for the regulations of bioavailability [2, 3].

Bioequivalence study is being performed to establish therapeutic efficacy of a particular drug product based on pharmacokinetic parameters (pK) where pK parameters of a test drug is compared with an innovator or reference drug.

Pharmacokinetics is the application of mathematical calculation and modeling techniques to the time course of absorption, distribution, metabolism, and excretion of drugs in the body. It is primarily concerned with the analysis of concentration and rate of drug availability to the required receptor site. Analysis of plasma samples will target concentration of drug as time progresses, resulting in the production of a 'plasma drug concentration-time curve'. Plasma drug concentration time curve can be obtained after a single oral dose of a drug by measuring concentration of drug in plasma samples taken at various intervals of time and plotting the concentration of drug in plasma vs corresponding time at which plasma samples were collected. BE study can be coined as the comparative pharmacokinetic study, where the bioequivalence was established based on the following parameters of test and innovator drug product-- maximum plasma concentration (Cmax), time to reach the maximum plasma concentration (Tmax), half-life (t½): time taken for the plasma concentration to fall by 50% and area under the plasma concentration curve (AUC): a calculation to assess the bodies total exposure to a drug over a given time [4, 5].

Pharmacokinetics is the application of mathematical calculation and modeling techniques to the time course of absorption, distribution, metabolism, and excretion of drugs in the body. It is primarily concerned with the analysis of concentration and rate of drug availability to the required receptor site.

Sample analysis will target concentration of drug as time progresses, resulting in the production of a 'plasma drug concentration-time curve'. Plasma drug concentration time curve can be obtained after a single oral dose of a drug by measuring concentration of drug in plasma samples taken at various intervals of time and plotting the concentration of drug in plasma (Y-axis) vs corresponding time at which plasma samples were collected (X-axis). Pharmacokinetics parameters calculated from this graph are Maximum plasma concentration (Cmax), Time to maximum plasma concentration (Tmax), Area under the plasma concentration curve (AUC): a calculation to assess the body's total exposure to a drug over a given time, Half-life ($t_{1/2}$): time taken for the plasma concentration to fall by 50%.

When a volunteer no I consumes a test drug (say one tablet of Montelukast 10mg) it goes to stomach and often the pharmacological action through ADME (absorption, distribution, metabolism and excretion) the drug reaches into the systemic circulation.

With the increase of time, the concentration increases and reaches its maximum (Cmax at time Tmax) along the absorption phase (A) and afterwards the concentrations of drug declines along the Elimination phase (B) as illustrated below.

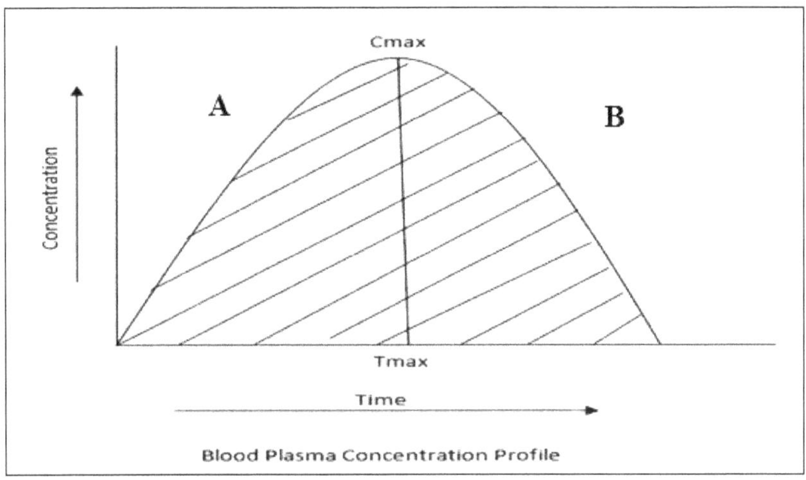

Similarly the same volunteer I will produce the plasma concentration profile as given below when he has consumed a reference drug (Spiromont-Montelukast 10mg).The PK parameters(Cmax, tmax, AUC) resulted from these two profiles of Test and reference products of 16/24 volunteers are compared by statistical analysis to establish bioequivalency.

Any drug which has come to India within four years has to be approved by CDSCO-HQ, New Delhi, Govt. of India based on BA/BE study and or CT reports along with other necessary documents. Besides New Drugs, the following are the areas where Bioavailability/Bioequivalence study reports are essential as per regulatory requirements.

1. FDC (Fixed Dose Combination) as per approved lists
2. SR (Sustained Release) Products
3. As per the Gazette Notification [GSR-327(E) dated 3rd April, 2017] regarding BCS Classification [6].
4. As directed by regulatory Authority

Many generic products are available in the markets and it has become a public concern that these products are similar to that of innovator in terms of safety and efficacy. Therefore a valid evaluation is necessary to guarantee the quality of these products. These intensified the importance of such studies to the pharmaceutical industry, contract research organizations (CRO) as well as regulators. For export market, BA/BE Study Report of the drug is one of the essential component in the dossier.

Table 1 Biopharmaceutical Classification System (BCS)

BCS	Permeability	Solubility	Remarks
Class I	High	High	Those compounds are well absorbed and their absorption rate is usually higher than excretion
Class II	High	Low	The bioavailability of those products is limited by their solvation rate. A correlation between the in vivo bioavailability and the in vitro solvation can be found
Class III	Low	High	The absorption is limited by the permeation rate but the drug is solvated very fast. If the formulation does not change the permeability or gastro-intestinal duration time, then class I criteria can be applied.
Class IV	Low	Low	Those compounds have a poor bioavailability. Usually they are not well absorbed over the intestinal mucosa and a high variability is expected.
It is mandatory to submit the result of bioequivalence study for obtaining the Marketing license from CDSCO for the drugs categorized as BCS class-II and IV for the Indian drug manufacturers			

Presently 82 CROs which are approved by FDA, India had been rendering services to a huge number of Pharma Industries in India and abroad. In spite of the potential job opportunities in the field of Bio-analytical Studies as well as Bioequivalence Studies, the trained manpower is not sufficiently available especially in Eastern Region. It is felt that more & more BA/BE Centre's have to be established to fulfill the present demand of the country.

References

1. India Brand Equity Foundation (IBEF). An initiative of the Ministry of Commerce & Industry, Government of India. Reports on Indian Pharmaceutical Industry.
   https://www.ibef.org/industry/pharmaceutical-india.aspx.

2. Midha KK, McKay G. Bioequivalence; Its History, Practice, and Future. The AAPS Journal. 2009 (11) 4, 664-670. DOI: 10.1208/s12248-009-9142-z.

3. US FDA Guidance for Industry: Bioavailability and Bioequivalence Studies Submitted in NDAs or INDs—General Considerations.
   https://www.fda.gov/downloads/drugs/guidancecomplianceregulator yinformation/guidances/ucm389370.pdf.

4. Galgatte UC, Jamdade VR, Aute PP, Chaudhari PD. Study on requirements of bioequivalence for registration of pharmaceutical

products in USA, Europe and Canada. Saudi Pharmaceutical Journal: SPJ. 2014; 22 (5):391-402.
DOI:10.1016/j.jsps.2013.05.001.

5. Central Drugs Standard Control Organization (CDSCO), Ministry of Health and Family Welfare, Government of India. Guidelines for Bioavailability and Bioequivalence studies. file:///K:/BA-BE%20Paper/BE%20Guidelines%20Draft%20Ver10%20March%20 16,%2005.pdf.

6. G.S.R. 327(E) dated 3rd April, 2017. Ministry of Health and Family Welfare, Govt. of India, New Delhi.
http://www.cdsco.nic.in/writereaddata/GSR%20327(E)%20Dated%2 003_04_2017.pdf.

Chapter 2

Essential Components required for BA/BE Study Centre

As per the Indian regulatory guidelines (CDSCO), following documents are required during submission of application for the approval of the BA/BE study center.

Document required for approval of BA-BE center

1) Covering letter.

2) Name and address of the organization to be registered along with its telephone no. , fax no. and email address.

3) Name and address of the proprietors/partners/directors.

4) An organogram of the organizational including brief CV of Key personnel.

5) Status of organization as legal identity (Recent registration certificate/ Memorandum and article association of firm).

6) Brief profile of specific activity/services undertaken by the organization including facilities, resources and infrastructure.

7) List of equipment in the firm.

8) List of staff in firm.

9) List of SOP's and SOP for Informed Consent process with Inform Consent Form.

10) Lay out of facility.

11) All details of Ethics Committee including composition of ethics committee.

12) All major tie ups for ancillary services like ambulance, hospital etc.

(http://www.cdsco.nic.in/writereaddata/Document-required-for-approval-of-BA-BE-center.pdf.).

In this chapter, essential components of a BA/BE study center are elaborated. Major departments are tabulated as follows:

- ❖ Bioanalytical Laboratory
- ❖ Clinical Pharmacology Unit (CPU)

❖ Documentation, Data Management and Archival Unit

❖ Administrative Unit

Bio-Analytical Laboratory

The Laboratory should be equipped with essential state-of-art instrumental facilities for the analysis of drug in plasma as listed in Table 2.

Table 2 List of Major & Minor Equipments required in a BA/BE Study Centre

Sl.	Instrument
1	HPLC with UV detector
2	HPLC with PDA detector
3	LC-MS/MS (liquid chromatography mass spectrometry)
4	Automatic off line Tablet Dissolution Apparatus with auto sampler
5	Deep Freezer (-20°C) in AU
6	Deep Freezer (-20°C) in CPU
7	Cold Centrifuge (-20°C) 20000rpm in CPU and AU
8	Centrifuge
9	Electronic Weighing balance
10	pH meter
11	UV-VIS Spectrophotometer
12	Hot Air Oven
13	Ultra sonic Bath
14	Water Bath (Digital)
15	Vortex Mixture
16	Millipore water System for HPLC
17	Sphygmomanometer (Blood Pressure) M/C, ECG/ Nebulizer / oxygen Saturation Meter etc
18	Pipettes, Water Baths
19	Humidity Chambers (IP Storage)
20	Plasma Extraction Unit (LLE)
21	Evaporator (Speedovac) for Plasma extraction
22	Other minor equipments to handle plasma samples

It is to be noted that all the instruments should be properly validated and calibrated by authorized company preferably NABL accredited. The user logbooks have to be kept for each and every instrument. Necessary standard operating procedures (SOPs) need to be displayed in front of the instrument. The approximate space required is illustrated in Fig.1.

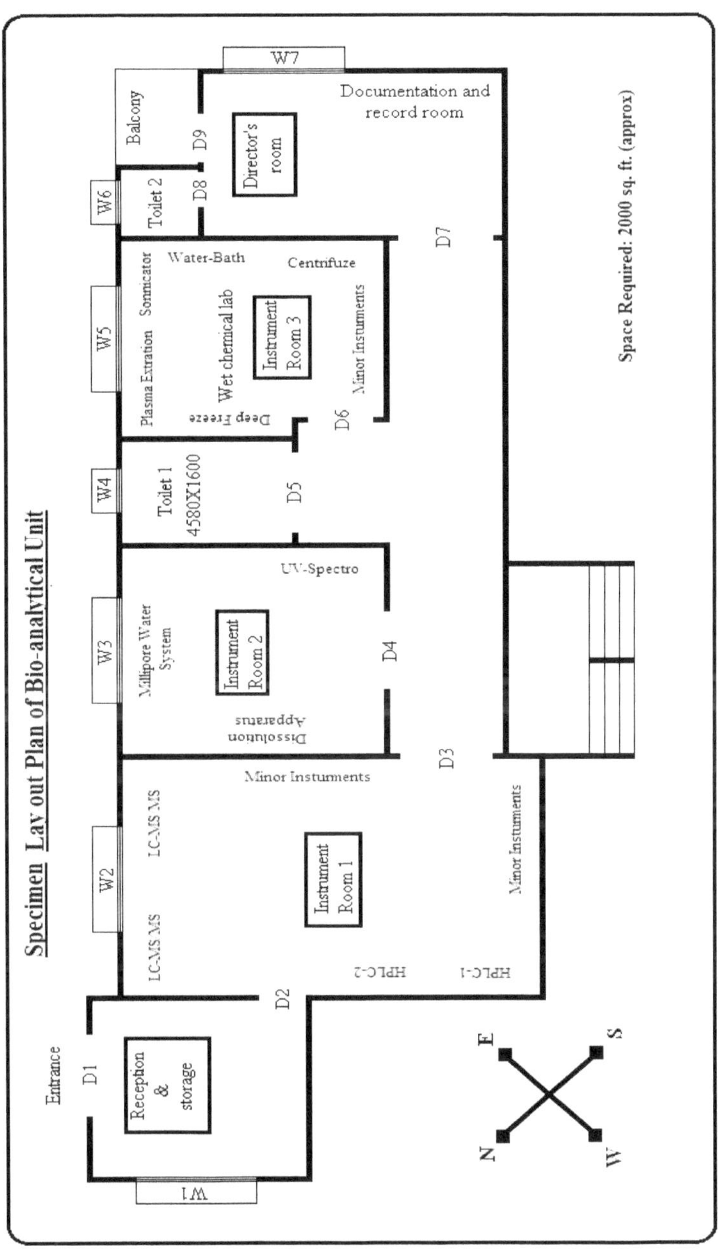

Figure 1 Specimen Layout Plan of Bio-analytical Unit

A Bio-analyst should have the experience & expertise to extract the drug component from plasma and its analysis by HPLC or LC-MS/MS (Liquid Chromatography and Mass spectrometry).

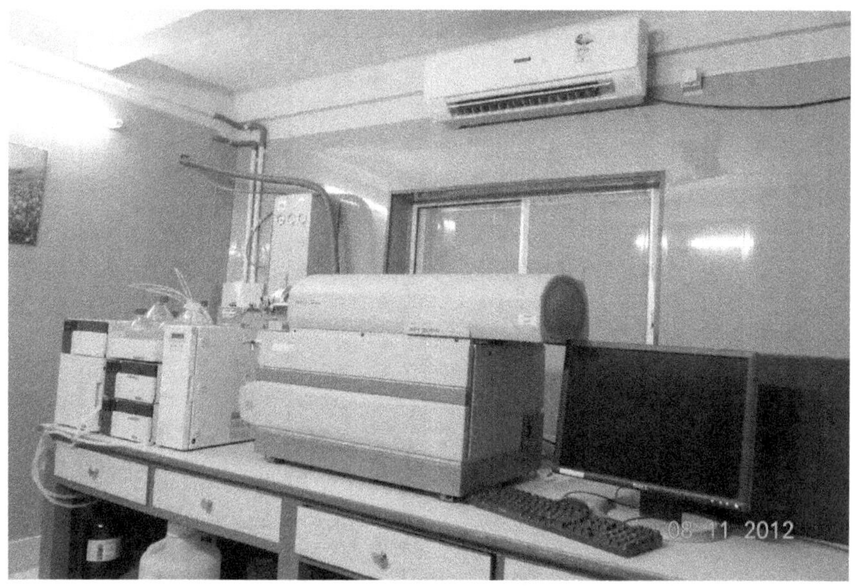

LC-MS/MS Instrument (API-200)
(Courtesy: TAAB Biostudy Services)

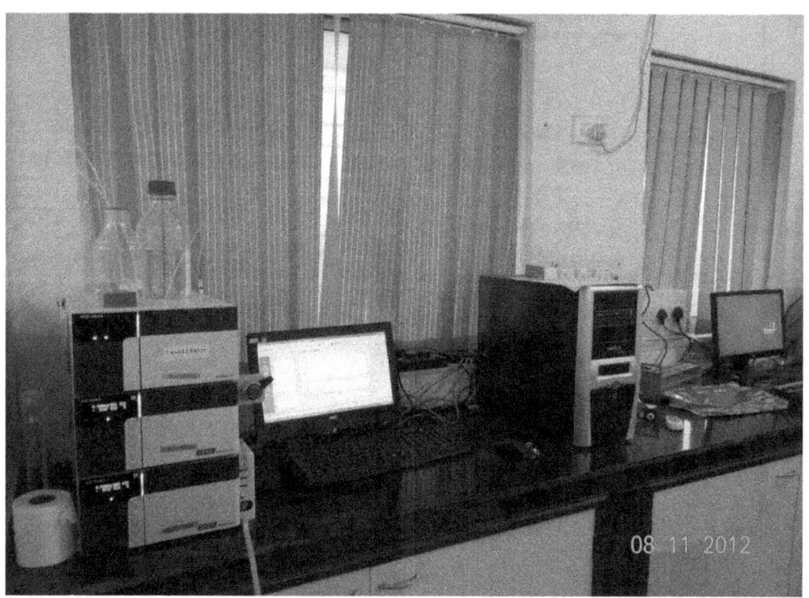

HPLC (with PDA detector)

(Courtesy: TAAB Biostudy Services)

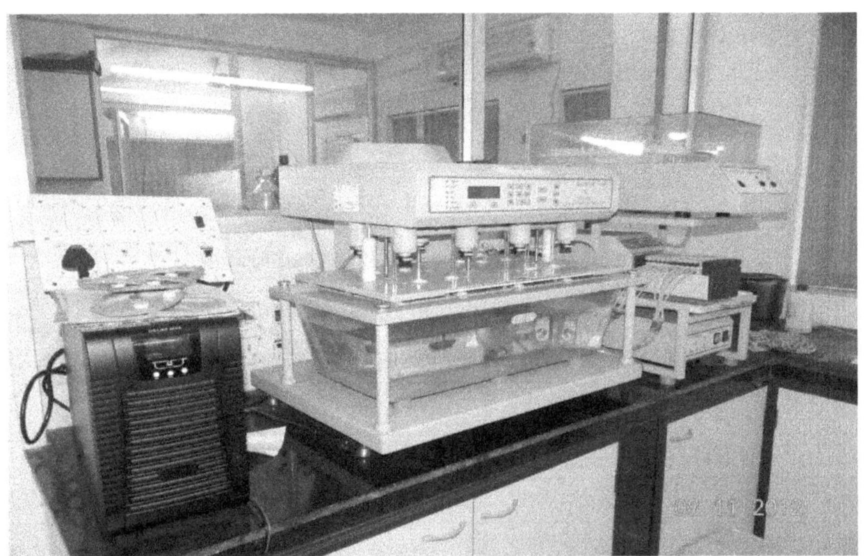

Dissolution Apparatus with Auto sampler

(Courtesy: TAAB Biostudy Services)

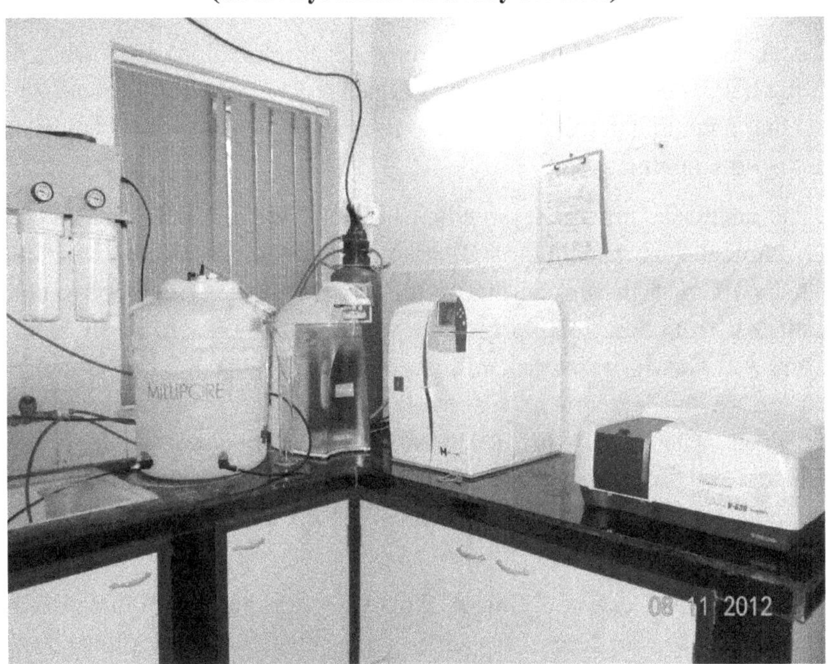

Millipore and Milli-Q Water System

(Courtesy: TAAB Biostudy Services)

For conducting Bio-analytical study, the proposed manpower and their qualification requirements are given in the Organogram of BA/BE study center in Table 3.

Table 3 Key persons with their qualification and responsibilities in Analytical Unit

Sl.	Designation	Qualification
1	Head, Bio-analytical	B. Pharm /M. Sc./ M. Pharm / Ph. D
2	Lab In-charge	B. Pharm/ M. Pharm/ Ph. D
3	Head, Quality Assurance	M. Pharm/ Ph. D
4	Research Scientist	B. Sc/ B. Pharm/ M. Sc./
5	Research Assistant	M. Pharm /Ph. D
6	Consultant	M. Pharm/Ph. D
Please note: Relevant Bioanalytical Experience and Training is essential for the Staffs		

Clinical Pharmacology Unit (CPU)

Clinical facility should have minimum accommodation of 16 to 24+2 healthy human volunteers in air-conditioned rooms with TV, Carrom board and other amenities for enjoyment and relaxation as well as ICU facility for one to two volunteers.

The necessary emergency medicines should be available in the CPU. The Clinical Pharmacologist (Doctor), Phlebotomists, Nurse and other related staff must be present during the BA/BE Study. The blood samples withdrawn from the volunteers have to be centrifuged to separate drug plasma and should be stored in a deep freezer (-20°C). There should be requisite tie-up, agreement for waste disposal of syringe cottons and needles etc. The temperature & Humidity recording logbooks according to regulatory requirements (within 25°C and 50% RH) have to be maintained. The food supply and laundry services should also be recorded as per regulatory requirement.

The major and essential tie-ups should be with the nearby hospital and nursing home to take care of any emergency situation of the volunteers due to AE (Adverse Event) or SAE (Serious Adverse Event) during conduction of BA/BE study. The tentative staff requirement with their qualification is illustrated in Table-4 and the specimen layout plan of CPU is given in Figure 2.

Table 4 Key persons with their qualification and responsibilities in Clinical Pharmacological Unit

Sl.	Designation	Qualification
1	Requisite number of Clinical Pharmacologist/ Principal Investigator (PI)	MBBS, MD (Pharmacology)/ DM (Clinical Pharmacology)
2	Study Coordinator	M. Pharm, Ph. D
3	Asst. Study Coordinator	B. Pharm/M. Pharm
4	Consultant Pathologist	MBBS, MD (Pathology)
5	Requisite number of Phlebotomist	DMLT
6	Nurse	Diploma/ Certificate
7	2Nos of Assistant Supervisor	B. Sc./12th
8	Peon	10th
9	Sweeper	

Please note: Relevant Experience and Training is essential for the Staffs

Table 5 List of Major & Minor Equipments required in CPU

Sl.	Instrument
1	Sphygmomanometer (B.P. M/C)
2	ECG Machine
3	Weighing Machine
4	Height Measuring Instrument
5	Cold Centrifuge (-20°C) 20000rpm
6	Deep Freezer (-20°C) in CPU
7	Humidity Chambers (IP Storage)
8	Pipettes
9	Pulse Oximeter
10	Nebulizer Machine
11	Oxygen Cylinder
12	Other Major and Minor Equipments

Note: All the machines/ instruments must be calibrated

It is to be noted that ICU facility with at least one bed is essential in clinical pharmacology unit as per regulatory requirements. Some essential medicines should be kept in sufficient quantity at the clinical pharmacology unit to handle any emergency situation during the conducting of clinical study on healthy volunteers.

List of Probable Essential Medicines Required at Clinical Pharmacological Unit

- Ringer Lactate Sol^n for Injection 500ml
- Normal Saline (0.9% w/v) Inj. IP 500ml
- DNS (0.9% and 5%) Injection IP 500ml
- Dextrose (5%) Injection 500ml
- Infusion Set
- Dispo Van Syringe (20ml)
- Dispo Van Syringe (10ml)
- Dispo Van Syringe (5ml)
- Dispo Van Syringe (2ml)
- Feeding Catheter
- IV Cannula
- Top Winged Infusion Set
- BD Neoflon
- Avil 25 Tablet
- Calpol 650mg Tablet
- Decolic Tablet
- Aciloc RD Tablet
- Combiflam Tablet
- Gelusil Tablet
- Gelusil Liquid
- Lanoxin Tablet 0.25mg
- Sorbitrate 10mg
- Calmpose Injection 2ml
- Deriphyllin Injection 2ml
- Water for Injection
- Zofer MD-4 Tablets
- Domstal Tablets
- Ondem MD-4 Tablets
- Rantac Injection 2ml
- Voveran Injection 1ml
- Decdan Injection 2ml
- Zofer MD-8 Tablets
- Reglan Injection
- Pantoprazole (Pan) Injection 40mg
- Decolic Injection 2ml
- Phenergan Injection 2ml
- Zofer Injection
- Asthalin Inhaler
- Rantac Tablet
- Budecort 0.5 mg

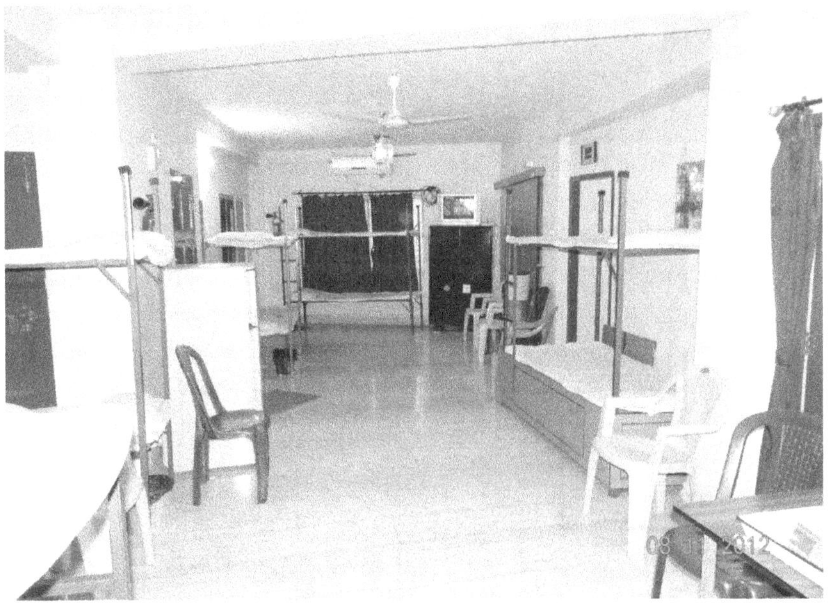

Partial view of the Clinical Pharmacological Unit (CPU)

(Courtesy: TAAB Biostudy Services)

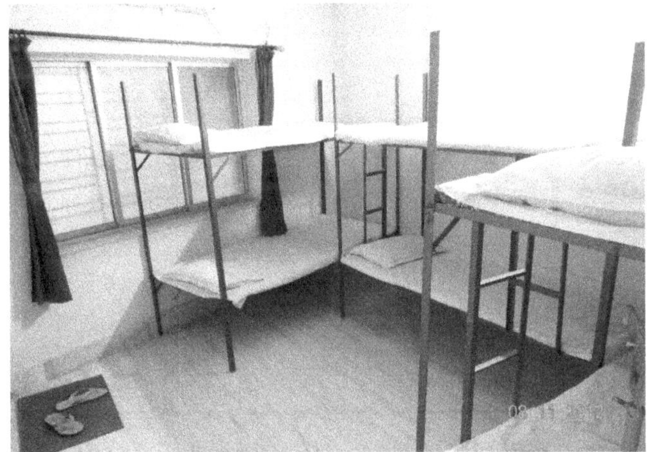

Volunteer Bed's at Clinical Pharmacological Unit (CPU)

(Courtesy: TAAB Biostudy Services)

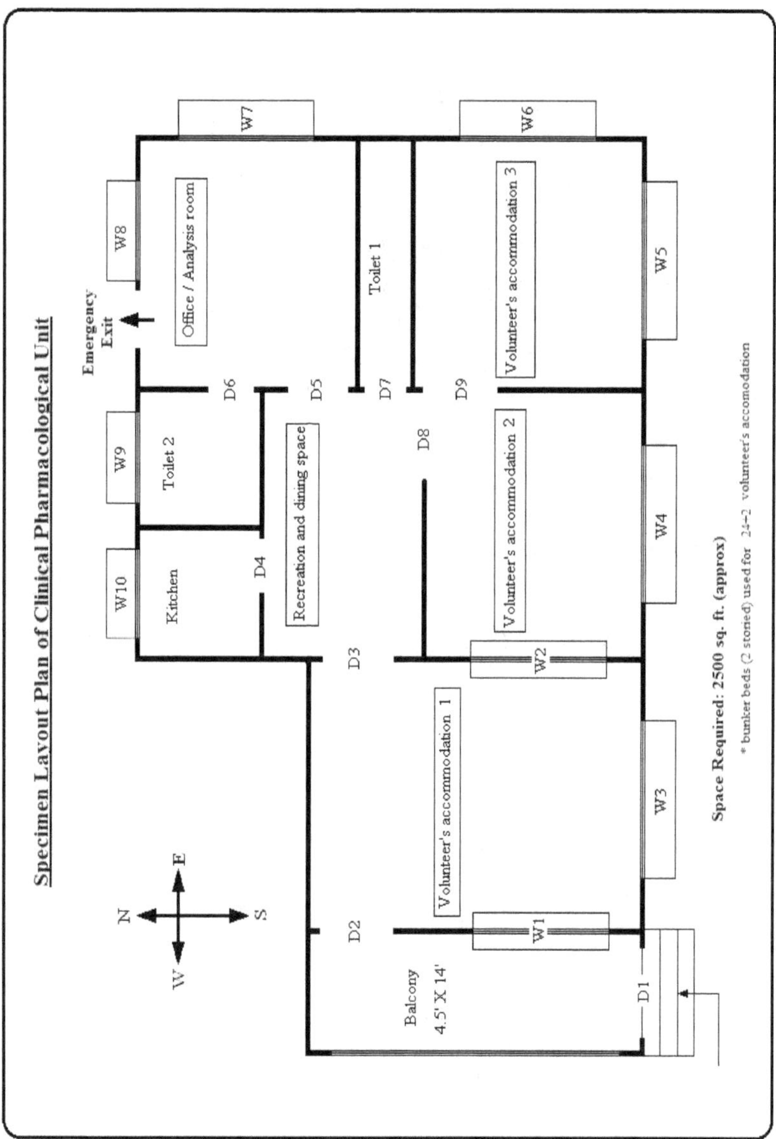

Figure 2 Specimen Layout Plan of Clinical Pharmacological Unit

Documentation, Data Management & Archiving Unit

The Bioanalytical unit will be sending the plasma concentration data to documentation unit where the technical staff will be engaged to evaluate the pharmacokinetic parameters (C_{max}, T_{max}, AUC_{0-t}, $AUC_{0-\infty}$, Kel & $t_{1/2}$) etc of these test and reference drug products. These results are further stimulated to prove bioequivalency based on statistical analysis (SAS or Win Nolin) with the help of Biostatistician.

The tentative staff requirement along with their qualification is stated in Table 6.

Table 6 Key persons with their qualification and responsibilities in Documentation Unit

Sl.	Designation	Qualification
1	Documentation & Compilation (In charge)	B. Sc/ B. Pharm/M. Pharm
2	Assistant Office Executive	MA/BA/B.Sc/M.Sc
3	Research Scientist	M. Sc., PGDCRRA /M. Pharm
4	Research Scientist	B. Pharm, PGDCRRA
5	Consultant Biostatistician	B.Sc/ M.Sc (Stat/Math)
6	Biostatistician	Ph.D, M. Sc. (Math)
7	Research Assistant	B.Sc., PGDCRRA
Please note: Relevant Experience and Training in compilation is essential for the Staff		

Administrative Unit

The tentative staff requirement along with their qualification is stated in Table 7.

Table 7 Key persons with their qualification and responsibilities in Administrative Unit

Sl.	Designation	Qualification
1	Office In-charge/ HR	MBA/ B.Sc/ M.Sc
2	Accountant	B.Com
3	Chartered Accountant	M.Com, CA

Standard Operating Procedures

Specific and elaborate instructions in a SOP format is very much required for each and individual operations in the CRO. The SOP is required for the instrumental operations as well as the processes without instruments. The major standard operating procedures (SOP's) is listed below in Table 8.

Table 8 Major Standard Operating Procedures (SOP's) Required in BA/BE Study Centre

Sl.	Title of the SOP
HR Department	
1	SOP for staff screening and recruitment
Quality Assurance Department (QA)	
2	SOP for use and maintenance of standard operating procedure
3	SOP for quality assurance unit and its functions

Table 8 *Contd...*

Sl.	Title of the SOP
4	SOP for documentation of training and qualification of employees
5	SOP for Preparation, approval, distribution, amendment, storage and archival
6	SOP for record keeping, reporting, storage and retrieval of data
Clinical Pharmacology Department (CPU)	
7	SOP for volunteer screening and recruitment and management of ineligible volunteers
8	SOP for bringing volunteers in the clinical unit and recycling the volunteers
9	SOP for pre-study physical and clinical examination of volunteers
10	SOP for collection and handling of biological samples
11	SOP for transportation of biological samples from clinical laboratory to analytical laboratory
12	SOP for administration of oral dosage forms of the drug to human subjects during BA/BE study
13	SOP for handling of subject check-in and check-out
14	SOP for adverse event monitoring ,recording and reporting
15	SOP for distribution of meals to the study subjects
16	SOP for obtaining written informed consent
17	SOP for study approval process by ethical committee
18	SOP for control of outsourcing process
19	SOP for cannulation of the study subjects
20	SOP for recording of vital signs of subjects
21	SOP for recording temperature and relative humidity
22	SOP for disposal of biological waste materials
23	SOP for operation of high speed (Elektrocraft) cold centrifuge machine
24	SOP for operation of 12 lead electrocardiograph (Cardiart 108T) machine
25	SOP for operation of 12 lead electrocardiograph (Vega 3 Channel ECG Machine)
26	SOP for drug sample handling and accountability
27	SOP for operation of low temperature freezer (-20°C)
28	SOP for compensation of injury or serious adverse event for subjects participating in the bioequivalence study
29	SOP for subject withdrawal or dropout from the BA/BE study
30	SOP for coding and decoding of the biological samples
31	SOP for Recording of Video for the Informed Consent Procedure During Inclusion of Volunteers in the BA/BE Study
32	SOP for Signal Detection & Risk Management in Pharmacovigilance
Analytical Department (AU)	
33	SOP for receipt of biological samples from Clinical Unit
34	SOP for operation of high speed (Eltek) cold centrifuge machine

Table 8 *Contd...*

35	SOP for operation of Eltek centrifuge machine
36	SOP for operating the high performance liquid chromatography (Jasco, Japan)
37	SOP for operating and maintenance of precision weighing balance
38	SOP for operating the automatic off line tablet dissolution apparatus with auto sampler
39	SOP for operating and calibration of pH meter
40	SOP for operating the high performance liquid chromatography (Knaur, Germany)
41	SOP for operation of Deep (low temperature) freezer (-20°C)
42	SOP for recording temperature and relative humidity at different areas in the analytical laboratory
43	SOP for method validation and analysis of volunteer plasma samples
44	SOP for operating the UV-Visible Spectrophotometer (Jasco, Japan)
45	SOP for operating the high performance liquid chromatography (Schimadzu, Japan)
46	SOP For Liquid Chromatography -Mass Spectrometry / Mass Spectrometry (API-2000) (LC-MS/MS-I)

A standard SOP format is attached herewith as a model.

Format for Standard Operating Procedure (Sop)

TITLE: STANDARD OPERATING PROCEDURE FOR PRE-STUDY PHYSICAL AND CLINICAL EXAMINATION OF VOLUNTEERS	
SOP NO.: XXX/XX/XX/01	DOC.NO.: XXX/XX/01
VERSION NO: XX	EFFECTIVE DATE:
SUPERSEDES: XXX/XX/XX/01, VERSION: 01	PAGE NO: 1 OF 3

Revision History

SOP Revision	Page(s)	Description of change(s)	Superseded Document
XXX/XX/XX/01			

Purpose	:	The purpose of this SOP is to describe the standard format and methodology at this site. The procedure is intended to meet FDA federal regulations (21 CFR 50, 54, 56, 312, and 314, 812 and 814) as well as Good Clinical Practice Guidelines.
Scope	:	This SOP applies to the Physicians at Clinical Pharmacology Units to assure the service at XXXX.
Objective	:	The objective of this SOP is to define the procedure for pre-study physical examination of volunteers during volunteer screening and recruitment for Bioequivalence Study in the Clinical Pharmacology Unit (CPU) of XXXX.
Responsibilities	:	<ul><li>Physicians in the Clinical Pharmacology Department of XXXXX are responsible for physical examination and documentation as per Good Clinical Practice (GCPs).</li><li>The Principal Investigator and the site clinical research staff are hereafter responsible for any SOP additions or revisions, as well as complying with site SOPs involving clinical trials.</li><li>SOPs must be approved by the Director.</li></ul>

PREPARED BY	CHECKED BY	APPROVED BY	DATE OF ISSUE:
Study Coordinator	Clinical	Technical Advisor	
			DATE OF REVISION:
XXXXX	XXXXX	XXXXXX	

TITLE: STANDARD OPERATING PROCEDURE FOR PRE-STUDY PHYSICAL AND CLINICAL EXAMINATION OF VOLUNTEERS

SOP NO.: XXX/XX/XX/01	DOC.NO.: XXX/XX/01
VERSION NO: XX	EFFECTIVE DATE:
SUPERSEDES: XXX/XX/XX/01, VERSION: 01	PAGE NO: 2 OF 3

Procedure

A. One Case Report Form containing the pre-study physical and clinical examination will be issued whenever an individual will reach at Clinical Pharmacology Unit of XXXXXX for screening purpose to participate in the bioequivalence study.

B. Taking rest for more than 30 minutes, the Name and Serial number of volunteer will be recorded in the Case Report Form.

C. Age, height and weight of the volunteer will be recorded. BMI will be calculated according to the following formula

$$BMI = \frac{Weight(kg)}{Height^2\left(mt^2\right)}$$

D. Once the BMI check is found within the limit, volunteers will be later called by the physician and the pulse rate, diastolic and systolic blood pressure with the help of calibrated blood pressure measuring instrument; body temperature with calibrated thermometer, respiratory rate will be recorded and documented in the Case Report Form. [The acceptable limit of pulse rate is 72 to 90/min, Blood pressure 100 to 150 mm Hg systolic and 50 to 90 mm Hg diastolic supine, Body temperature < 99.0°F, Respiratory rate 12 to 15/min].

E. Physical Examinations will be performed for different body organs by the physician and if they found fit for participation in the biostudy, they will be sent to the phlebotomist to give 10 mL blood sample for routine haematology [Total WBC count, differential count (Neutrophyl, Lymphocyte, Monocytes, Eosinophil and Basophil and haemoglobin], biochemistry [blood glucose, urea, bilirubin (direct, total), total protein, albumin, globulin, A/G ratio, SGPT, alkaline phosphatase, creatinine, cholesterol, Na^+ and K^+ and serology (HIV, Hepatitis and Syphilis) test.

F. Upon receipt of the volunteer blood test results, the volunteer will be evaluated for their eligibility in the biostudy.

G. If the post study safety evaluation is to be done for the subjects completing the clinical study, the vital signs will be checked along with the Clinical Examinations [including haematology {Total WBC count, differential count (Neutrophyl, Lymphocyte, Monocytes, Eosinophil and Basophil) and haemoglobin}, biochemistry {blood glucose, urea, bilirubin (direct, total), total protein, SGPT, alkaline phosphatase, creatinine, cholesterol}] will be performed.

PREPARED BY	CHECKED BY	APPROVED BY	DATE OF ISSUE:
Study Coordinator	Clinical Pharmacologist	Technical Advisor	
			DATE OF REVISION:
XXXXX	XXXXX	XXXXXX	
TITLE: STANDARD OPERATING PROCEDURE FOR PRE-STUDY PHYSICAL AND CLINICAL EXAMINATION OF VOLUNTEERS			
SOP NO.: XXX/XX/XX/01		DOC.NO.: XXX/XX/01	
VERSION NO: 02		EFFECTIVE DATE:	
SUPERSEDES: XXX/XX/XX/01, VERSION: 01		PAGE NO: 3 OF 3	

H. The subjects will be asked to come after five days of the completion of the clinical study. Any subject who develops any adverse event or clinically significant abnormal laboratory test values will be evaluated, and will be treated and /or followed up until the symptoms or values return to normal or acceptable levels, as judged by the Investigator /Doctor.

References

❖ FDA federal regulations (21 CFR 50, 54, 56, 312, and 314, 812 and 814)

❖ Good Clinical Practice Guidelines

❖ CDSCO Guidelines

PREPARED BY	CHECKED BY	APPROVED BY	DATE OF ISSUE:
Study Coordinator	Clinical Pharmacologist	Technical Advisor	
			DATE OF REVISION:
XXXXX	XXXXX	XXXXXX	

Chapter 3

Ethical Perspectives

Ethics Committee including its Composition

Biomedical research in India is expected to incorporate three essential ethical safeguards, in addition to following applicable national and local laws: conformation to the declaration of Helsinki [1] approval of research protocol and supervision of the research process by an ethical committee, and signed informed consents from all the willing participants of this study.

Further, ethical approval from the concerned ethics committee is mandatory before carrying out biomedical research. Bioethics is defined as "A systemic study of the moral dimensions including moral vision, decision, conduct and policy of the life sciences and health care, employing a variety of ethical methodologies in an interdisciplinary setting".

Biomedical research ethics involves:

- ❖ Sponsored inputs about; study design, study outcomes, sample size and study duration
- ❖ Informed consent procedures
- ❖ Compensation for trial related injury
- ❖ Effective monitoring (Pre study, Post study and during study)
- ❖ Ensuring confidentiality, Justice and Fairness
- ❖ Vulnerable subject protection

In India, the classic regulatory guidelines to be followed for biomedical research[2] is 'Ethical guidelines for biomedical research on human participants' published by Indian Council of Medical Research (ICMR of 2006).

Early in 2013, the Drugs & Cosmetics Rules-1945 had a new addition of sub-clause 122DD after its predecessor 122DC. This has been incorporated as per the Gazette Notification [GSR 72 (E)] dated 8th February 2013 [3]. Incorporation of rule 122DD mandates that every Ethics Committee in India whether it is institutional or independent, must be registered at the office of the Drugs Controller General of India before it is granted approval for a clinical trial. The definition of this rule as CDSCO stated is "An Ethics Committee is a committee comprising of scientific, medical, non-medical and non-scientific members, whose responsibility is to ensure the protection of the rights, safety and well-being of human subjects involved in a clinical trial and it shall be responsible for reviewing and approving the protocol, the suitability of the investigators, facilities, methods and adequacy of information to be used for obtaining and documenting informed consent of the study subjects and adequacy of confidentiality safeguards."

Prior to conducting any BA/BE Study the protocol has to be approved by the respective Independent Bioethics Committee which must be registered by the licensing authority (CDSCO, Govt. of India).

The composition of Ethics committee with their designations is illustrated in table 9 according to Appendix VIII of Schedule Y of Drugs and cosmetics Act 1940 [4, 5].

Table 9 Composition of a CDSCO Approved Independent/Institutional Ethics Committee

Designation	Number of Persons Required
Chairman	1 (outside of the institute/organization)
Member Secretary	1
Clinician	2
Clinical Pharmacologist	2
Medical Scientist	1
Lawyer	1
Layman	1
Social Worker	1
Total No of Members	**15 maximum**
Please note that one female representation is mandatory	

CDSCO approval copy of a registered independent ethics committee along with the rules and regulations for functioning of the ethics committee are elaborated as a ready reference.

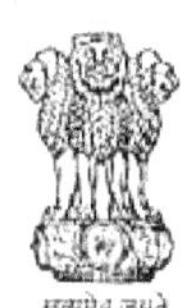

Government of India
Ministry of Health & Family Welfare
Directorate General of Health Services
Office of Drugs Controller General (India)
Central Drugs Standard Control Organization

सत्यमेव जयते

FDA Bhawan, Kotla Road,
New Delhi – 110 002, India
Dated:

To

The Chairman
Independent Bioethics Committee

Kolkata- 700032, West Bangal
India

Sub: - Ethics Committee Re-registration No.   ssued under Rule 122DD
       of the Drugs & Cosmetics Rules1945.

Sir/Madam,

Please refer to your application submitted to this Directorate for the Re-registration of Ethics Committee.

Based on the documents submitted by you, this office hereby re-registers the
COMMITTEE situated at
KOLKATA- 700032, WEST BANGAL, INDIA with Re-registration Number   as per the provisions of Rule 122DD of the Drugs and Cosmetics Rules, 1945 subject to the following conditions:

1. The re-registration shall be in force from 16.08.2016 to 15.08.2019, unless it is sooner suspended or cancelled.

2. The Ethics Committee shall review and approve only the study protocols and related documents of Bioavailability/Bioequivalence studies of the approved drug molecules and also carry ongoing review of such studies.

3. The Ethics Committee shall review and accord its approval to Bioavailability/Bioequivalence studies and also carry ongoing review of such studies at appropriate intervals, as specified in Schedule Y and the Good Clinical Practice Guidelines for Clinical Trials in India and other applicable regulatory requirements for safeguarding the rights, safety and well being of the trial subjects.

4. In the case of any serious adverse event occurring during Bioavailability/Bioequivalence studies, the Ethics Committee shall analyze and forward its opinion as per procedures specified under APPENDIX XII of Schedule Y.

5. The Ethics Committee shall allow inspectors or officials authorized by the Central Drugs Standard Control Organization to enter its premises to inspect any record, data or any document related to Bioavailability/Bioequivalence studies and provide adequate replies to any query raised by such inspectors or officials, as the case may be, in relation to the conduct of Bioavailability/Bioequivalence studies.

6. The licensing authority shall be informed in writing in case of any change in the membership or the constitution of the ethics committee takes place.

7. All the records of the ethics committee shall be safely maintained after the completion or termination of the study for not less than five years from the date of completion or termination of the trial (Both hard and soft copies).

8. If the Ethics Committee fails to comply with any of the conditions of registration, the Licensing Authority may, after giving an opportunity to show cause why such an order should not be passed, by an order in writing stating the reasons therefore, suspend or cancel the registration of the Ethics Committee for such period as considered necessary.

9. This registration shall be in force for a period of three years from the date of issue, unless it is sooner suspended or cancelled.

10. Ethics Committee shall consist of not less than seven members and is subject to a maximum of 15. One among its members, who is from outside the institute, shall be appointed as chairman, one member as a Member Secretary and rest of the members shall be from Medical, Scientific, Non Medical and Non-scientific fields including lay public.

11. The committee shall include at least one member whose primary area of interest or specialization is Non-scientific and at least one member who is independent of the institution besides; there should be appropriate gender representation on the Ethics Committee.

12. The Ethics committee can have as its members, individuals from other Institutions or Communities, if required.

13. Members should be conversant with the provisions under Schedule Y, Good Clinical Practice Guidelines for clinical trials in India and other regulatory requirements to safeguard the rights, safety and well-being of the trial subjects.

14. For review of each protocol the quorum of Ethics Committee shall be at least five members with the following representations:
    I.   Basic medical scientist (preferably one pharmacologist)
    II. Clinician
    III. Legal expert
    IV. Social scientist or representative of non-governmental voluntary agency or philosopher or ethicist or theologian or a similar person.
    V.   Lay person from community

15. The members representing medical scientist and clinicians should have Post graduate qualification and adequate experience in their respective fields and aware of their role and responsibilities as committee members.

16. As far as possible, based on the requirement of research area such as HIV, Genetic disorder, etc., specific patient group may also be represented in the Ethics Committee.

17. There should be no conflict of interest. The members shall voluntarily withdraw from the Ethics Committee meeting while making a decision on an application which evokes a conflict of interest which may be indicated in writing to the Chairman prior to the review and be recorded so in the minutes. All members shall sign a declaration on conflict of interest.

18. Subject experts or other experts may be invited to the meetings for their advice. But no such expert shall have voting rights.

19. This certificate is issued to you on the basis of declaration/ submission by you and that registration is sought for Independent Ethics Committee.

20. Ethics Committee should review such number of protocols of Bioavailability/Bioequivalence studies of approved drug molecules which should be commensurate to the infrastructure and facilities available with them.

21. Status report of the functioning of the Ethics Committee should be submitted to the CDSCO headquarters and concerned zonal office on quarterly basis.

22. The details of funding support and amount of honorarium, if any, payable to the ethics committee members should be defined in the Standard Operating Procedure (SOP) of the committee and records to this extent shall be maintained.

23. Ethics committee should have dedicated office with required infrastructure and supporting staff. SOP's for funding of the Ethics committee in order to support their operations must be maintained. The records of income & expenditure of Ethics Committee shall be maintained for review and inspection

24. Funding mechanisms for the Ethics Committee to support their operations should be designed to ensure that the committees and their members have no financial incentive to approve or reject particular studies.

25. SOP's for funding of the Ethics committee in order to support their operations must be maintained. The records of income & expenditure of Ethics Committee shall be maintained for review and inspection.

26. The Chairman of Ethics Committee shall enter into MOU with head of institution, that necessary support and facilities and independence will be provided to Ethics Committee and their records will be maintained as long as required.

27. Ethics Committee may undertake the review and monitoring of clinical trial protocols of other investigator(s) and site(s) who do not have their IEC, subject to the condition that the other sites are within the loco- regional and community settings similar to that of the registered Ethics committee. The approving ethics committee must be willing to accept their responsibilities for the study at such trial site(s) and the trial site(s) willing to accept such an arrangement.

28. Ethics Committee shall review and approve the suitability of the investigator and trial site for the proposed trial. The ethics committee shall undertake proper causality assessment of SAE's with the help of subject experts where required, for deciding relatedness and compensation, as per condition no (4) mentioned above.

Joint Drugs Controller (I) & Licensing Authority

Dossier submission for the Ethical Approval

The CRO/ Principal Investigator have to apply to the Chairman of the Ethics Committee for consideration of the study protocol and related documents. Generally following documents are needed at the time of the application for after application submission to the ethics committee:

- ❖ Protocol
- ❖ Informed Consent Form in English and/or vernacular language
- ❖ Patient/ Subject Information Sheet
- ❖ Investigator's undertaking
- ❖ Principal investigator's CV.
- ❖ Case report form
- ❖ Investigator's Brochure
- ❖ Insurance policy for participation and for serious adverse events occurring during the study participation
- ❖ Regulatory Permission Letter (if available)

The dossier will be received by the Chairman/ Secretary at least 7 to 10 days before the next scheduled date of meeting. A copy of the same will be distributed by the Secretary to all the members. Ethics Committee may invite the principal investigator or any person(s) specialized in a particular field who may provide special review of selected research protocols, if needed. Such person(s) generally have no voting power. Ethics approval usually issued upon every protocol found satisfactory as per the regulatory guidelines. A sample copy of the ethical approval issued by the HURIP Independent Bioethics Committee for a BA/BE study is furnished here as a ready reference [6, 7].

References

1. World Medical Association. The Declaration of Helsinki [Accessed on 25th September 2013]. Available from: http://www.wma.net/en/30publications/10policies/b3.

2. Ethical guidelines for biomedical research on human participants. New Delhi: Indian Council of Medical Research, 2006 [Accessed on 3rd January 2013]. Available from:

   http://icmr.nic.in/ethical_guidelines.pdf.

3. Amendment to the Drugs & Cosmetics Rules-1945, Gazette Notification [GSR 72 (E)] dated 8th February 2013 [Accessed on 19th October 2013]. Available from:
   http://cdsco.nic.in/html/G.S.R%2072(E)%20dated%2008.02.2013.pdf.

4. Central Drugs Standard Control Organization (CDSCO), Drugs and Cosmetics Rules, 1945 [Accessed on 25thSeptember2013]. Available from: http://cdsco.nic.in/html/D&C_Rules_Schedule_Y.pdf.

5. Shubhasis Dan, Balaram Ghosh, Bapi Gorain and T K Pal. "Mandatory Registration of the Research Ethics Committees in India". Applied Clinical Research, Clinical Trials & Regulatory Affairs, 2014, 1, 88-92.
   [DOI: 10.2174/2213476X019991408181112854].

6. CDSCO Registration Letter. Hurips Bioethics Committee, Kolkata-700032, West Bengal, India (ECR/103/Indt/WB/2013).

7. SOPs of the HURIP Independent Bioethics Committee, Kolkata, West Bengal.

To be printed on Ethics Committee Letterhead

To   Date: XXXX
Dr. XXXXX
Clinical Pharmacologist Principal Investigator
TAAB Biostudy Services
Jadavpur, Kolkata-32

Subject: Ethics committee approval of protocol for Bioequivalence Studies.

Dear Dr. XXXX.
The HURIP Independent Bioethics Committee reviewed and discussed your application to conduct the BA BE Study of the following drug.

Sl.	Study Title	Protocol No. & Date
1.	A Randomized, open label, two treatment, two period, two sequence, single dose, crossover, comparative, oral bioavailability study of (Study Drug) manufactured by (Name and address of the Sponsor) with marketed samples of (Reference Product) manufactured by (Name and address of the manufacturer of Reference Product) in 16 – 2 healthy, adult human male subjects under fasting conditions.	XXXX & XXXX

The following documents were reviewed:
- Trial protocol
- Patient Informed Consent Form
- Translation for Patient Informed Consent Forms (in Vernacular Languages)
- Patient Information Sheet
- Investigator's CV & MRC
- Investigator's undertaking
- Regulatory Permission Letter (If Available)

The study will be conducted at the (address of the CPU of the CRO).

The following members of HURIP Independent Bioethics Committee were present at the meeting held on (date and time) in office of HURIP (Office Address). (Names and designations of the members present.

Protocol bearing protocol number XXXXX and study related documents have been approved by the members of the Independent Ethics Committee. We approve the study to be conducted in its present form. HURIP Independent Bioethics Committee expects to be informed about the progress of the study, any SAE occurring in the course of study, any changes in the protocol or informed consent form and asked to be provided a copy of the final report.

Yours sincerely,

....   -----------------------------------
Secretary,   Chairman,
HURIP Independent Bioethics Committee   HURIP Independent Bioethics Committee.

1 of 1

Chapter 4

Pre-requisites for Conducting BA/BE Studies

In the previous chapter the facilities required for BA/BE studies and ethical perspectives have been discussed. It is also to be noted that the BA/BE study has to be carried out in a CDSCO approved CRO under the guidance of the Local Regulator (i.e. Ethics Committee).

To initiate any study the CRO (Contract Research Organization) have to follow the following steps.

❖ **Agreement**

An agreement of CDA (Confidential Non-disclosure agreement) and Research Service Agreement (Financial Agreement) between the CRO and Sponsor have to be signed.

❖ **Protocol**

The CRO will prepare the protocol in consultation with Clinical Pharmacologist (MBBS, MD) and Study Coordinator as per regulatory requirements and in agreement with the sponsor. The sponsor will be providing the details of the IP (Investigational Products) of both Test and Reference drug and API for BA/BE study.

❖ **Ethics Committee Approval**

The CRO (Bioequivalence Study Centre) will submit the protocol in its standard format to EC. The CDSCO registered Independent Bioethics Committee will review and scrutinize protocol towards its approval. The Ethics Committee will issue one approval letter to the respective CRO in favor of Principal Investigator (Clinical Pharmacologist).

NOC/Import License/Test License by DCGI (Drugs Control General of India)-The Sponsor will submit the protocol along with the other documents to DCGI for its approval to get NOC for domestic market and Import License for Export market. A specimen copy of NOC is enclosed herewith.

❖ **IP (Investigational Products)**

Once the NOC and Import License is obtained from DCGI office New Delhi, the sponsor will provide the necessary drug products

(Test and Reference) and API (Active Pharmaceutical Ingredients) with COA (Certificate of Analysis) to the CRO with covering letter. The CRO will maintain a record of these IP and API.

❖ **Clinical Study (Period I and Period II)**

Now the CRO is in the position to finalize the dates for clinical study on healthy human volunteers (16/24 numbers) in consultation with the principal Investigator according to approved protocol and SOP of the CRO.

In case of the foreign reference samples or BE study for export purpose, the CRO has to apply for the Import License for the examination, test and analysis purpose though CDSCO-SUGAM portal. All study related documents like protocol, EC approval, details of the test and reference products along with justification of quantity, country of import etc. have to be uploaded online. A sample copy of the cover letter along with approval (form-11) has been attached for ready reference.

List of Attachments

- Specimen copy of DCGI NOC (permission)

- Specimen copy of Import License to Conduct BA/BE Study

References

1. Central Drugs Standard Control Organization (CDSCO), Directorate General of Health Services, Ministry of Health & Family Welfare, Govt. of India, SUGAM-An e-Governance solution for CDSCO (Sugam Portal).
   https://cdscoonline.gov.in/CDSCO/homepage;jsessionid=8B2E7A636 9D6F401180497F081BCE8C7.

2. Central Drugs Standard Control Organization.
   http://cdsco.nic.in/forms/Default.aspx.

Specimen DCGI NOC for conducting BA/BE study

<table>
<tr><td>4385/03.</td><td>File No.04-24/2   0-DC (Pt.   )
Directorate General of Health Services
Office of Drugs Controller General (India)
(FDC Division)</td><td>Tele. No. : 011-23236965
Fax No.   : 011-23236973</td></tr>
</table>

FDA Bhawan, Kotla Road
New Delhi-110002
Dated: 2 9 MAR 2012

To,

<u>Subject</u>:   **Permission to conduct Bioequivalence study with the . . . . -Regarding.**

<u>BE NOC No.</u>: BE-Drugs/16/2012

Sir,

Please refer to your letter no. ████████████████ dated 20.01.2012   on   the   subject mentioned above. This Directorate has no objection to your conducting bioequivalence study with

as per study protocol No. 12/11/163 submitted to this Directorate subject to the following information shall be provided in the report:

1. Date of commencement and conclusion of the study.
2. Names and addresses of the volunteers who participated in the study.
3. Copy of consent letters of the volunteers.
4. Copy of Ethical Committee's approval.

You are requested to conduct comparative *in vitro* dissolution study and submit the report along with updated stability study data as per schedule Y requirements duly signed by the competent person alongwith report of BE study.

In case any unusual, unexpected or serious adverse reaction is observed during study, the same should be immediately communicated.

You are also requested to follow ethical aspects of the study as described "Ethical Guidelines for Biomedical Research on Human participant" published by ICMR, New Delhi and "Good Clinical Practice Guidelines" issued by this Directorate and to obtain Ethical Committee clearance of the institute where the trial is being conducted before initiation of the study.

One of your competent technical persons should be present during conduct of the study.

In case of study related injury of death, you will provide complete medical care as well as compensation for the injury or death and statement to this effect should be incorporated in the Informed Consent Form. Further in case of such injuries or death, the details of compensation provided should be intimated to this Directorate.

Yours faithfully,

Drugs Controller General (India)

Cover letter (Import License to Conduct BA/BE Study)

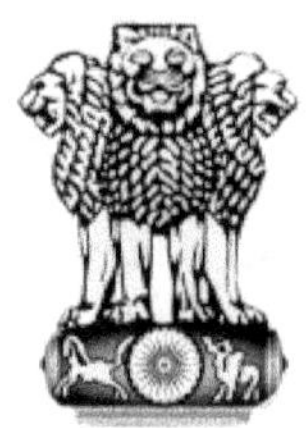

GOVERNMENT OF INDIA
CENTRAL DRUGS STANDARD CONTROL
ORGANISATION (East Zone)

(Directorate General of Health Services)
Ministry of Health & Family Welfare
O/o the Dy. Drugs Controller (I),Nizam Palace, 1st MSO
Building
7th Floor (Eastern Side),234/4, A.J.C. Bose Road
Kolkata - 700020 (West Bengal)
Phone No.: (033) 2287-0513, 2280-1391
Fax No.: (033) 2281-3806
E-Mail : cdscoez@cdsco.nic.in

F.No. TL/EZ/18/00002

Dated: 24-JUL-2018

To

M/s

Name and Address of CRO

Sir,

With reference to your application No. TL/Form12/EZ/2018/5629 dated 18-JUL-2018, please find enclosed herewith the 'licence for examination, test and analysis' bearing No. TL/EZ/18/00002 under the provisions of Drugs and Cosmetic Act and Rules to import the drug/drugs mentioned therein. Kindly acknowledge receipt of this letter and its enclosures.

Yours faithfully,

DEPUTY DRUGS CONTROLLER (I)
Licensing Authority

Copy together with a copy of Import License No. TL/EZ/18/00002
Forwarded for information to:-
• All port offices

Permission Letter/ Form-11 (Import License to Conduct BA/BE Study)

Form 11

[See Rule 33]

LICENCE TO IMPORT DRUGS FOR THE PURPOSES OF EXAMINATION, TEST OR ANALYSIS

Number of Licence: TL/EZ/18/00002

I, **Designated Person of the CRO**, of **Name & Address of the CRO** Kolkata, West Bengal - 700032 is hereby licensed to import from United States the drugs specified below for the purposes of examination, test or analysis at M/s **Name & Address of the CRO** or in such other places as the licensing authority may from time to time authorize.

2. This licence is subject to the conditions prescribed in the Rules under the Drugs and Cosmetics Act, 1940.

3. This licence shall, unless previously suspended or revoked, be in force for a period of three year from the date specified below:

S.No.	Name of drugs and Brand Name	Class of Drug	Quantity which may be imported
1	Ursodeoxycholic Acid 300mg Capsules 300 milligram (mg) (Actigall 300mg Capsules)	For the treatment of patients with chronic cholestatic liver disease	50 Capsules (10)

Item(s) One (1) only
Not for any commercial purpose and to be used for clinical studies/trials i.e.
BA/BE for Export purpose & related testing only

Digital Signature

Date 24-JUL-2018

LICENSING AUTHORITY
Seal/Stamp

Conditions of Licence

1. The licensee shall use the substances imported under the licence exclusively for purpose of examination, test or analysis and shall carry on such examination, test or analysis in the place specified in the licence, or in such other places as the licensing authority may from time to time authorise.

2. The licensee shall allow any inspector authorized by the licensing authority in this behalf to enter, with or without prior notice, the premises where the substances are kept, and to inspect the premises, and investigate the manner in which the substances are being used to take samples thereof;

3. The licensee shall keep a record of, and shall report to the licensing authority, the substances imported under the licence, together with the quantities imported, the date of importation and the name of the manufacturer.

4. The licensee shall comply with such further requirements, if any, applicable to the holders of licences for examination, test or analysis as may be specified in any rules subsequently made under Chapter III of the Act and of which the licensing authority has given to him not less than one month's notice.

5. The drugs imported under this licence shall not be directed to or for Commercial Marketing including export purposes

6. The firm shall obtain No Objection Certificate from the Narcotics Commissioner of India, 19, The Mall Morar, Gwalior for the import of drugs under Narcotic Drugs and Psychotropic Substances Act and Rules, 1985.

Chapter 5

Methods to Conduct BE Study

In this chapter, methods were elaborated to conduct Bioequivalence study on 16 healthy human volunteers. BA/BE study of Montelukast orally disintegrating strips 10mg have been chosen as a model study. Before initiation of a BA/BE study, the CRO has to develop a study protocol. The study protocol along with the related documents *i.e.* ICF (Informed Consent Form), CRF (Case Record Form) etc have to be finalized and approved by the sponsor.

The study methods were divided in the following parts *i.e.*

Before Initiation of the Study

A. Preparation of Study Protocol

B. Ethics Committee and Regulatory Approval

Initiation of the Study (Clinical, Bio-analytical)

C. *Clinical Phase*: Single dose exposure of the test and reference products has to be carried out and the plasma samples as per the time points specified in the approved protocol have to be collected.

D. *Bio-Analytical Phase*: Method development and Method Validation as per approved protocol. Analysis of volunteer plasma samples and quantification of the amount of drug present in human plasma to evaluate PK parameters (Pharmacokinetic) is undertaken.

E. *Statistical Analysis, Documentation and Compilation Phase*: Statistical analysis of PK parameters has to be performed to prove bioequivalency of Test product in comparison with Reference product with the help of SAS or Win Nolin 5.1.3. After statistical evaluation final report along with related documents has to be compiled.

Model Study Protocol

A study protocol entitled "A Randomized, open label, two treatment, two period, two sequence, single dose, crossover, comparative, oral bioavailability study of Montelukast Orally Disintegrating Strip 10 mg manufactured by (name of the sponsor) with marketed samples of Spiromont 10 mg Orally Disintegrating Strip manufactured by (name of the company) In (number of volunteers) healthy, adult human male subjects under fasting conditions" has been explained as model protocol. Similarly a method development and method validation protocol for montelukast 10 mg has also been illustrated.

Protocol No.: xx/xx/xxx   **Status: Final; Version: 1.0**
This document contains confidential information which is the property of (Name of The Sponsor). It is intended for your internal use only. Do not copy, disclose, or circulate externally without written authorization.
Date: ....

Protocol Number: xx/xx/xxx

Version no. 1.0

Date:

PROTOCOL TITLE

A Randomized, open label, two treatment, two period, two sequence, single dose, crossover, comparative, oral bioavailability study of Montelukast Orally Disintegrating Strip 10 mg (each orally disintegrating strip containing montelukast sodium IP equivalent to montelukast 10 mg) manufactured by (name of the sponsor) with marketed samples of Spiromont 10 mg Orally Disintegrating Strip (each orally disintegrating strip containing montelukast sodium IP equivalent to montelukast 10 mg) manufactured by (name of the company) In 16+2 or 24+2 healthy, adult human male subjects under fasting conditions

Sponsor

(Name & Address)

CRO

(Name & Address)

Protocol No.: xx/xx/xxx   **Status: Final; Version: 1.0**

This document contains confidential information which is the property of (Name of The Sponsor). It is intended for your internal use only. Do not copy, disclose, or circulate externally without written authorization.

Date: ....

INVESTIGATOR'S DECLARATION

We, the undersigned have read and understood this protocol and hereby agree to conduct the study in accordance with this protocol and to comply with all requirements regarding the obligations of investigators and all other pertinent requirements of the International Conference on Harmonization (ICH) [Step 4] 'Guideline for Good Clinical Practice (GCP) E6 [R1].', Good Laboratory Practice (GLP), Amended version of Schedule Y [2005], Central Drugs Standards Control Organization CDSCO India, Indian Council on Medical Research (ICMR) Guidelines for Biomedical Research on Human Participants, Declaration of Helsinki and other regulatory requirements.

We agree to comply with all relevant Standard Operating Procedures (SOPs) required for the conduct of this study. We further agree to ensure that all associates assisting in the conduct of this study will be informed regarding their obligations.

Clinical Investigator

Signature	**Date**

Study Coordinator

Signature	**Date**

Director/Technical Advisor

Signature	**Date**

Protocol No.: xx/xx/xxx   **Status: Final; Version: 1.0**
This document contains confidential information which is the property of (Name of The Sponsor). It is intended for your internal use only. Do not copy, disclose, or circulate externally without written authorization.
Date: ....

SPONSOR'S DECLARATION

(To be printed on sponsor's letter head)

I, the undersigned have read and understood this protocol and hereby agree to have the study conducted in accordance with this protocol and to comply with all requirements regarding the obligations of the sponsor and all other pertinent requirements of the ICH Guidelines for Good Clinical Practice for conducting BA/BE studies.

If any of the volunteers subjected to physical injury or death because of study drug, *(Name of the Sponsor and address)* will provide complete medical assistance as well as compensation for the injury or death, as per The Government of India, Gazette Notification No. GSR 53 (E) dated 30.01.2013 and amended vide GSR 889 (E) dated 12.12.2014.

____

Signatory Authority

On behalf of the Sponsor and address   **Date:...............**

Protocol No.: xx/xx/xxx   **Status: Final; Version: 1.0**
This document contains confidential information which is the property of (Name of The Sponsor). It is intended for your internal use only. Do not copy, disclose, or circulate externally without written authorization.
Date: ....

PROTOCOL SYNOPSIS

Study Title	A Randomized, open label, two treatment, two period, two sequence, single dose, crossover, comparative, oral bioavailability study of Montelukast Orally Disintegrating Strip 10 mg (each orally disintegrating strip containing montelukast sodium IP equivalent to montelukast 10 mg) manufactured by **(name of the sponsor)** with marketed samples of Spiromont 10 mg Orally Disintegrating Strip (each orally disintegrating strip containing montelukast sodium IP equivalent to montelukast 10 mg) manufactured by (name of the company) In **16+2** or **24+2** healthy, adult human male subjects under fasting conditions
Objective	To compare the oral bioavailability montelukast Orally Disintegrating Strip 10 mg (each orally disintegrating strip containing montelukast sodium IP equivalent to montelukast 10 mg) manufactured by **(name of the sponsor)** with marketed samples of Spiromont 10 mg Orally Disintegrating Strip (each orally disintegrating strip containing montelukast sodium IP equivalent to montelukast 10 mg) manufactured by (name of the company) In **16+2** or **24+2** healthy, adult human male subjects under fasting conditions
Trial Design	A randomized, open label, two treatment, two period, two sequence, single dose, crossover bioequivalence study under fasting conditions.
Subjects	**16+2** or **24+2** healthy, adult, human, male subjects.
Screening Procedures	Demographic data, medical and medication histories, physical examination, height, weight, vital signs, hematology, biochemistry and serology will be done at screening.
Housing	Housing from at least 11 hr prior to drug administration until after the 24 hr blood sampling.
Treatments	**Test [A2]:** Montelukast orally disintegrating strip 10 mg (each orally disintegrating strip containing Montelukast Sodium IP equivalent to Montelukast 10 mg) manufactured by **(Name of the Sponsor).**
	Reference [A1]: Spiromont 10 mg orally disintegrating strip (each orally disintegrating strip containing Montelukast Sodium IP equivalent to Montelukast 10 mg) manufactured by **(Name of Company).**
Drug Administration	As per the randomization schedule, single ODS (Orally Disintegrating Strip) of either Test or Reference product will be orally administered to

Protocol No.: xx/xx/xxx   **Status: Final; Version: 1.0**
This document contains confidential information which is the property of (Name of The Sponsor). It is intended for your internal use only. Do not copy, disclose, or circulate externally without written authorization.
Date: ....

	each subject in each period in sitting posture after an overnight fast of at least 10 hr. Both the test product and reference product will be given to the volunteers without water initially and after complete disintegration of the strip, 240 ml of water will be provided. The subjects will receive a standardized meal 4.0 hr post-dose. Water will be permitted *ad libitum* except for 1.0 hr before and until 1.0 hr post dose.
Blood Sampling	In each of the study period, 11 blood samples will be collected in 5 mL K_2EDTA vacutainers via an indwelling catheter placed in one of the forearm vein. Blood samples will also be collected by direct venipuncture during ambulatory blood sampling visit as well as wherever necessary for any practical reason. The pre-dose blood sample will be collected within a period of 1hr prior to the drug administration. The post-dose blood samples will be collected at 0.5, 1.0, 2.0, 2.5, 3.0, 4.0, 6.0, 8.0, 12.0 and 24.0 hrs. All the blood samples for a particular sample time point, will be centrifuged under refrigeration at 3500 rpm and 4°C for 10 min. The resulting plasma will be separated and stored in suitably labeled polypropylene tubes at $-20 \pm 5°C$ for pending assay. The total volume of blood drawn including the volume necessary for the laboratory tests [screening and safety sample], PK analysis and the volume of blood discarded before each blood draw will be about 129 mL per subject for the entire study.
Subject Monitoring	Clinical examination and vital signs measurements [blood pressure, pulse rate, respiration rate and oral temperature] will be recorded at check-in and check-out and Vital signs will also be recorded before dosing of investigational products. Clinical examination and measurement of vital signs may also be carried out at any time during the conduct of the study if the Investigator/Doctor feels necessary. In case of abnormality in vital signs during pre-dose vitals recording, medical opinion will be taken whether to dose the subject or not. During recording of vital signs, each subject will be asked about his wellbeing.
Post-study Procedures	Physical examination, vital signs will be done at the end of the clinical part of the study as safety evaluation.
Washout	At least 7 days gap between two consecutive dosing days will be maintained.

Protocol No.: xx/xx/xxx   **Status: Final; Version: 1.0**

This document contains confidential information which is the property of (Name of The Sponsor). It is intended for your internal use only. Do not copy, disclose, or circulate externally without written authorization.

Date: ....

Pharmacokinetic Parameters	C_{max}, T_{max}, AUC_{0-t}, $AUC_{0-\infty}$, K_{el} and $t_{1/2}$
Analytical Methods	Montelukast in plasma will be quantified using validated LC-MS/MS method.
Statistical Methods	Statistical analyses will be done using SAS version 9.1.3/ WinNonlin version 5.3. Analysis of Variance [ANOVA] for log-transformed pharmacokinetic parameters [C_{max}, AUC_{0-t} and $AUC_{0-\infty}$] will be performed. Ratio and 90% Confidence Interval for ratio and power for log-transformed pharmacokinetic parameters $-C_{max}$, AUC_{0-t} and $AUC_{0-\infty}$ will be calculated.
Standards for Bioequivalence	The calculated 90% Confidence Interval should fall within 80 to 125% for the Test/Reference ratios for AUC_{0-t}, $AUC_{0-\infty}$ and C_{max} to conclude bioequivalence.

Protocol No.: xx/xx/xxx   **Status: Final; Version: 1.0**
This document contains confidential information which is the property of (Name of The Sponsor). It is intended for your internal use only. Do not copy, disclose, or circulate externally without written authorization.
Date: ....

FACILITIES OF THE CRO ALONG WITH ADDRESS

CLINICAL UNIT   ....

ANALYTICAL LABORATORY   ....

DATA ANALYSIS   ....

SPONSOR   ....

PATHOLOGICAL LABORATORY ....

BIO-WASTE MANAGEMENT   ....

CATERING SERVICES   ....

IEC SERVICES   ....

EMERGENCY MANAGEMENT   ....

Protocol No.: xx/xx/xxx   **Status: Final; Version: 1.0**
This document contains confidential information which is the property of (Name of The Sponsor). It is intended for your internal use only. Do not copy, disclose, or circulate externally without written authorization.
Date: ....

TABLE OF CONTENTS

- **Protocol Title**
- **Investigator's Declaration**
- **Protocol Synopsis**
- **Facilities**
- **Table of Contents**
- **Abbreviations**

1.0	**Background and Pharmacokinetics**		
2.0	**Objective**		
3.0	**Study Design**		
4.0	**Subject Selection and Restriction**		
5.0	**Clinical Procedures**		
6.0	**Data Analysis**		
7.0	**Clinical Supplies**		
8.0	**Ethical Considerations**		
9.0	**Analytical Procedures**		
10.0	**Treatment of Time Point Deviation**		
11.0	**Procedure for Reporting Any Deviation(s) from Original Statistical Plan**		
12.0	**Study Report and Documents**		
13.0	**Supplementary Documentation**		
14.0	**Archives**		
15.0	**Direct Access to Source Data/Documents**		
16.0	**Quality Control and Quality Assurance**		
17.0	**Publication**		
18.0	**Changes in Protocol**		
19.0	**References**		
20.0	**List of Appendices**		
	•Appendix I	Declaration of Helsinki	
	•Appendix II	ICF, Subject Information Sheet (English)	
	•Appendix III	ICF, Subject Information Sheet (Bengali)	
	•Appendix IV	Schedule of study event	
	•Appendix V	Case Record Form	
	•Appendix VI	Table of Study Diet	
	•Appendix VII	Investigator's undertaking	
	•Appendix VIII	Serious adverse event form	
	•Appendix IX	Utilization Breakup	

Protocol No.: xx/xx/xxx   **Status: Final; Version: 1.0**

This document contains confidential information which is the property of (Name of The Sponsor). It is intended for your internal use only. Do not copy, disclose, or circulate externally without written authorization.

Date: ....

ABBREVIATIONS

ADR	Adverse Drug Reaction
AE	Adverse Event
ANOVA	Analysis of Variance
AUC_{0-t}	The area under the plasma concentration versus time
$AUC_{0-\infty}$	Area under the plasma concentration versus time curve
BMI	Body Mass Index
bpm	Beats per Minute
CDSCO	Central Drugs Standards Control Organization
CI	Confidence Intervals
C_{max}	Maximum measured plasma concentration
cm	Centimeter
COA	Certificate of Analysis
CFR	Code of Federal Regulation
CRF	Case Record Form
CV	Curriculum Vitae
DCGI	Drugs Controller General of India
EDTA	Ethylene diamine tetra acetic acid
GCP	Good Clinical Practice
GLP	Good Laboratory Practice
Hb	Hemoglobin
HDL	High Density Lipoprotein
HIV	Human Immunodeficiency Virus
HPLC	High Performance Liquid Chromatography
h/hr	Hour
ICF	Informed Consent Form
ICH	International Conference on Harmonization
ICMR	Indian Council of Medical Research
IEC	Independent Ethics Committee
IRB	Institutional Review Board
K_{el}	Elimination rate constant
kg	Kilogram
LC-MS	Liquid Chromatography-Tandem Mass spectrometry

Protocol No.: xx/xx/xxx   **Status: Final; Version: 1.0**
This document contains confidential information which is the property of (Name of
The Sponsor). It is intended for your internal use only. Do not copy, disclose, or
circulate externally without written authorization.
Date: ....

LFT	Liver Function Test
LH	Luteinizing Hormone
ln/Ln	Natural Logarithm
LOQ	Limit of Quantification
max	Maximum
MBBS	Bachelor of Medicine Bachelor of Surgery
MD	Doctor of Medicine
mg	Milligram
min	Minimum
Min	Minute
mL	Milliliter
mmHg	Millimeter of Mercury
M.Sc.	Master of Science
NAV	Not available
PK	Pharmacokinetic
QA	Quality Assurance
RBC	Red Blood Cell
RPM	Revolutions per minute
SAE	Serious Adverse Event
SD	Standard Deviation
sec	Second
SEM	Standard Error of the Mean
SOP	Standard Operating Procedure
$t_{1/2}$	Elimination half life
T_{max}	Time to maximum concentration
USFDA	United States Food and Drug Administration
USP	United States Pharmacopeia
WBC	White Blood Corpuscle
WHO	World Health Organization
WMA	World Medical Association
%CV	Percentage Coefficient of Variation

Protocol No.: xx/xx/xxx   **Status: Final; Version: 1.0**
This document contains confidential information which is the property of
(Name of The Sponsor). It is intended for your internal use only. Do not
copy, disclose, or circulate externally without written authorization.
Date: ....

1.0   Background and Pharmacokinetics

Description: Montelukast sodium is a hygroscopic; optically active; photolabile; white-colored (or whitish) powder It is a potent; orally active compound with anti-inflammatory properties that significantly improves asthmatic inflammation parameters. It binds with great affinity and selectivity to CysLT1 receptors over other pharmacologically important receptors of the respiratory tract; such as the prostanoid; cholinergic; or β-adrenergic receptors. Montelukast potently inhibits physiological actions of LTC4; LTD4; LTE4 leukotrienes at CysLT1 receptors without any agonist activity. Therefore; it is indicated for the prophylaxis and chronic treatment of asthma in adults and 12-month-old or older pediatric patients; and it helps to control the symptoms of seasonal and perennial allergic rhinitis. Montelukast sodium is described chemically as [R-(E)]-1-[[[1-[3-[2-(7-chloro-2-quinolinyl) ethenyl] phenyl]-3-[2-(1-hydroxy-1-methylethyl) phenyl] propyl] thio] methyl] cyclopropaneacetic acid, monosodium salt.

The empirical formula is $C_{35}H_{35}ClNNaO_3S$, and its molecular weight is 608.18. Montelukast sodium is freely soluble in ethanol, methanol, and water and practically insoluble in acetonitrile. The structural formula is:

The objective of this study will be to establish the bioequivalence of two Montelukast formulations; comparing the bioavailability of a single dose of Montelukast 10 mg Orally disintegrating strip(ODS) produced by **(Name of the Sponsor)** (Test Product) to a single dose of Spiromont 10mg ODS containing Montelukast 10 mg produced by (name of the Manufacturer) (Reference Product).

Protocol No.: xx/xx/xxx   **Status: Final; Version: 1.0**
This document contains confidential information which is the property of (Name of The Sponsor). It is intended for your internal use only. Do not copy, disclose, or circulate externally without written authorization.
Date: ....

Clinical Pharmacology

Mechanism of action: The cysteinyl leukotrienes (LTC4, LTD4, LTE4), are potent inflammatory eicosanoids released from various cells including mast cells and eosinophils. These important pro-asthmatic mediators bind to cysteinyl leukotriene (CysLT) receptors. The CysLT type-1 (CysLT1) receptor is found in the human airway (including airway smooth muscle cells and airway macrophages) and on other pro-inflammatory cells (including eosinophils and certain myeloid stem cells). CysLTs have been correlated with the pathophysiology of asthma and allergic rhinitis. In asthma, leukotriene- mediated effects include a number of airway actions, including bronchoconstriction, mucous secretion, vascular permeability, and eosinophil recruitment. In allergic rhinitis, CysLTs are released from the nasal mucosa after allergen exposure during both early- and late-phase reactions and are associated with symptoms of allergic rhinitis. Intranasal challenge with CysLTs has been shown to increase nasal airway resistance and symptoms of nasal obstruction. Montelukast sodium has not been assessed in intranasal challenge studies. The clinical relevance of intranasal challenge studies is unknown.

Montelukast is an orally active compound that improves parameters of asthmatic inflammation. Based on biochemical and pharmacological bioassays, it binds with high affinity and selectivity to the CysLT1 receptor (in preference to other pharmacologically important airway receptors such as the prostanoid, cholinergic, or β-adrenergic receptor). Montelukast potently inhibits physiologic actions of LTC4, LTD4, and LTE4 at the CysLT1 receptor without any agonist activity.

Pharmacodynamics: Montelukast causes inhibition of airway cysteinyl leukotriene receptors as demonstrated by the ability to inhibit bronchoconstriction due to inhaled LTD4 in asthmatic patients. Doses as low as 5 mg cause substantial blockage of LTD4-induced bronchoconstriction. In a placebo-controlled, crossover study (n = 12), montelukast sodium inhibited early and late-phase bronchoconstriction due to antigen challenge by 75% and 57% respectively.

Montelukast causes bronchodilation within 2 hrs of oral administration; these effects were additive to the bronchodilation caused by a β-agonist. Clinical studies in adults 15 yrs of age and older demonstrated there is no additional clinical benefit to montelukast doses above 10 mg once daily. This was shown in two chronic asthma studies using doses up to 200 mg once daily and in one exercise challenge study using doses up. The effect of

Protocol No.: xx/xx/xxx   **Status: Final; Version: 1.0**
This document contains confidential information which is the property of (Name of The Sponsor). It is intended for your internal use only. Do not copy, disclose, or circulate externally without written authorization.
Date: ....

montelukast sodium on eosinophils in the peripheral blood was examined in clinical trials in adults and paediatric (6 to 14 yrs of age) asthmatic patients. Montelukast sodium decreased mean peripheral blood eosinophil approximately 13% to 15% from baseline compared with placebo over the double-blind treatment periods. In patients with seasonal allergic rhinitis aged 15 yrs and older who received montelukast sodium, a median decrease of 13% in peripheral blood eosinophil counts was noted, compared with placebo, over the double-blind treatment periods.

Pharmacokinetics

Absorption: Montelukast is rapidly absorbed following oral administration. For the 10 mg film coated tablet, the mean peak plasma concentration (C_{max}) is achieved in 3 to 4 hrs (T_{max}) after administration in adults in the fasted state. The mean oral bioavailability is 64%. The oral bioavailability and C_{max} are neither influenced by a standard meal in the morning nor by a high fat snack in the evening. Safety and efficacy were demonstrated in clinical trials where the 10 mg film-coated tablet was administered in the evening without regard to the timing of food ingestion.

Distribution: Montelukast is more than 99% bound to plasma proteins. The steady-state volume of distribution of montelukast averages 8 to 11 liters. Studies in rats with radiolabeled montelukast indicate minimal distribution across the blood-brain barrier. In addition, concentrations of radiolabeled material at 24 hrs post dose were minimal in all other tissues.

Metabolism: Montelukast is extensively metabolized. In studies with therapeutic doses, plasma concentrations of metabolites of montelukast are undetectable at steady state in adults and pediatric patients. *In-vitro* studies using human liver microsomes indicate that cytochrome P450 3A4, 2C8 and 2C9 are involved in the metabolism of montelukast. CYP 2C8 appears to play a major role in the metabolism of montelukast at clinically relevant concentrations.

Elimination: The plasma clearance of montelukast averages 45 mL/min in healthy adults. Following an oral dose of radiolabeled montelukast, 86% of the radioactivity was recovered in 5 day fecal collections and <0.2% was recovered in urine. Coupled with estimates of montelukast oral bioavailability, this indicates montelukast and its metabolites are excreted almost exclusively via the bile.

In several studies, the mean plasma half-life of montelukast ranged from 2.7 to 5.5 hrs in healthy young adults. The pharmacokinetics of

Protocol No.: xx/xx/xxx   **Status: Final; Version: 1.0**
This document contains confidential information which is the property of (Name of The Sponsor). It is intended for your internal use only. Do not copy, disclose, or circulate externally without written authorization.
Date: ....

montelukast are nearly linear for oral doses up to 50 mg. No difference in pharmacokinetics was noted between dosing in the morning or in the evening. During once-daily dosing with 10 mg montelukast, there is little accumulation of the parent drug in plasma (~14%).

Non-Clinical Toxicology

Carcinogenicity, Genotoxicity, Impairment of Fertility: No evidence of tumorigenicity was seen in carcinogenicity studies of either 2 yrs in Sprague-Dawley rats or 92 weeks in mice at oral gavage doses up to 200 mg/kg/day or 100 mg/kg/day, respectively. The estimated exposure in rats was approximately 120 and 75 times the AUC for adults and children, respectively, at the maximum recommended daily oral dose. Montelukast demonstrated no evidence of mutagenic or clastogenic activity in the following assays: the microbial mutagenesis assay, the V-79 mammalian cell mutagenesis assay, the alkaline elution assay in rat hepatocytes, the chromosomal aberration assay in Chinese hamster ovary cells, and in the *in-vivo* mouse bone marrow chromosomal aberration assay. In fertility studies in female rats, montelukast produced reductions in fertility and fecundity indices at an oral dose of 200 mg/kg (estimated exposure was approximately 70 times the AUC for adults at the maximum recommended daily oral dose).

Use in Specific Populations

Pregnancy: There are no adequate and well-controlled studies in pregnant women. Because animal reproduction studies are not always predictive of human response, montelukast should be used during pregnancy only if clearly needed.

Teratogenicity: No teratogenicity was observed in rats and rabbits at doses approximately 100 and 110 times, respectively, the maximum recommended daily oral dose in adults based on AUCs.

Nursing Mothers: Studies in rats have shown that montelukast is excreted in milk. It is not known if montelukast is excreted in human milk. Because many drugs are excreted in human milk, caution should be exercised when montelukast is given to a nursing mother.

Geriatric Use: Of the total number of subjects in clinical studies of montelukast, 3.5% were 65 yrs of age and over, and 0.4% was 75 yrs of age and over. No overall differences in safety or effectiveness were observed between these subjects and younger subjects, and other reported clinical

Protocol No.: xx/xx/xxx   **Status: Final; Version: 1.0**
This document contains confidential information which is the property of (Name of The Sponsor). It is intended for your internal use only. Do not copy, disclose, or circulate externally without written authorization.
Date: ....

experience has not identified differences in responses between the elderly and younger patients, but greater sensitivity of some older individuals cannot be ruled out. The pharmacokinetic profile and the oral bioavailability of a single 10 mg oral dose of montelukast are similar in elderly and younger adults. The plasma half-life of montelukast is slightly longer in the elderly. No dosage adjustment in the elderly is required.

Paediatrics Use: The plasma concentration profile of montelukast following the administration of 10 mg film-coated tablet is similar in adolescent's $\geq$15 yrs old and young adults. The 10 mg film-coated tablet is recommended for use in patients' $\geq$15 yrs old.

Gender: The pharmacokinetics of montelukast is similar in males and females.

Race: Pharmacokinetic differences due to race have not been studied. In clinical studies, there do not appear to be any differences in clinically important effects.

Renal Impairment: Since montelukast and its metabolites are not excreted in the urine, the pharmacokinetics of montelukast was not evaluated in patients with renal insufficiency. No dosage adjustment is recommended in these patients.

Hepatic Impairment: Patients with mild to moderate hepatic insufficiency and clinical evidence of cirrhosis had evidence of decreased metabolism of montelukast resulting in approximately 41% higher mean montelukast area under the plasma concentration curve (AUC) following a single 10 mg dose. The elimination of montelukast is slightly prolonged compared with that in healthy subjects (mean half-life, 7.4 hrs). No dosage adjustment is required in patients with mild to moderate hepatic insufficiency. There are no clinical data in patients with hepatitis or severe hepatic insufficiency. No dosage adjustment is required in patients with mild-to-moderate hepatic insufficiency.

Interaction: Montelukast sodium may be administered with other therapies routinely used in the prophylaxis and chronic treatment of asthma, and in the treatment of allergic rhinitis. Although additional specific interaction studies were not performed, montelukast sodium was used concomitantly with a wide range of commonly prescribed drugs in clinical studies without evidence of clinical adverse interactions. These medications included thyroid hormones, sedative hypnotics, nonsteroidal anti-inflammatory agents, benzodiazepines and decongestants.

In-vitro studies have shown that montelukast is a potent inhibitor of CYP 2C8. However, data from a clinical drug-drug interaction study involving montelukast and rosiglitazone (a probe substrate representative of drugs primarily metabolized by CYP 2C8) in 12 healthy individuals demonstrated that the pharmacokinetics of rosiglitazone are not altered when the drugs are coadministered, indicating that montelukast does not inhibit CYP 2C8 *in-vivo*. Therefore, montelukast is not anticipated to alter the metabolism of drugs metabolized by this enzyme (*e.g.,* paclitaxel, rosiglitazone, repaglinide). Based on further in vitro results in human liver microsomes, therapeutic plasma concentrations of montelukast do not inhibit CYP 3A4, 2C9, 1A2, 2A6, 2C19, or 2D6. *In-vitro* studies have shown that montelukast is a substrate of CYP 2C8, 2C9, and 3A4. Data from a clinical drug-drug interaction study involving montelukast and gemfibrozil (an inhibitor of both CYP 2C8 and 2C9) demonstrated that gemfibrozil increased the systemic exposure of montelukast by 4.4-fold. Based on clinical experience, no dosage adjustment of montelukast is required upon coadministration with gemfibrozil. Based on in vitro data, clinically important drug interactions with other known inhibitors of CYP 2C8 (*e.g.,* trimethoprim) are not anticipated.

Indications: Montelukast is indicated in the treatment of asthma as add-on therapy in those patients with mild to moderate persistent asthma who are inadequately controlled on inhaled corticosteroids and in whom "as-needed" short acting beta-agonists provide inadequate clinical control of asthma. In those asthmatic patients in whom Montelukast is indicated in asthma, montelukast can also provide symptomatic relief of seasonal allergic rhinitis. Montelukast is also indicated in the prophylaxis of asthma in which the predominant component is exercise-induced bronchoconstriction. Montelukast is indicatesd in adults and adolescents from the age of 15yrs.

Contraindications: Montelukast are contraindicated in patients with hypersensitivity to the drug or any of its components.

Adverse Reactions

The following adverse reactions have been reported in post-marketing use:

- ***Blood and lymphatic system disorders:*** Increased bleeding tendency
- ***Immune system disorders:*** Hypersensitivity reactions including anaphylaxis, hepatic eosinophilic infiltration

Protocol No.: xx/xx/xxx   **Status: Final; Version: 1.0**
This document contains confidential information which is the property of (Name of The Sponsor). It is intended for your internal use only. Do not copy, disclose, or circulate externally without written authorization.
Date: ....

- ***Psychiatric disorders:*** Dream abnormalities including nightmares, hallucinations, psychomotor hyperactivity (including irritability, restlessness, agitation including aggressive behavior, and tremor), depression, insomnia

- ***Nervous system disorders:*** Dizziness drowsiness, paraesthesia/hypoesthesia, seizure

- ***Cardiac disorder:*** Palpitations

- ***Gastrointestinal disorders:*** Diarrhoea, dry mouth, dyspepsia, nausea, vomiting

- ***Hepatobiliary disorders:*** Elevated levels of serum transaminases (ALT, AST), cholestatic hepatitis

- ***Skin and subcutaneous tissue disorders:*** Angioedema, bruising, urticaria, pruritus, rash

- ***Musculoskeletal and connective tissue disorders:*** Arthralgia, myalgia including muscle cramps

- ***General disorders and administration site conditions:*** Asthenia/fatigue, malaise, oedema

Warning and Precaution

Acute Asthma: Montelukast sodium is not indicated for use in the reversal of bronchospasm in acute asthma attacks, including status asthmaticus. Patients should be advised to have appropriate rescue medication available. Therapy with montelukast sodium can be continued during acute exacerbations of asthma. Patients who have exacerbations of asthma after exercise should have available for rescue a short-acting inhaled β-agonist.

Concomitant Corticosteroid Use: While the dose of inhaled corticosteroid may be reduced gradually under medical supervision, montelukast sodium should not be abruptly substituted for inhaled or oral corticosteroids.

Aspirin Sensitivity: Patients with known aspirin sensitivity should continue avoidance of aspirin or non-steroidal anti-inflammatory agents while taking montelukast sodium. Although montelukast sodium is effective in improving airway function in asthmatics with documented aspirin sensitivity, it has not been shown to truncate bronchoconstrictor response to aspirin and other non-steroidal anti-inflammatory drugs in aspirin-sensitive asthmatic patients

Neuropsychiatric Events: Neuropsychiatric events have been reported in adult, adolescent, and pediatric patients taking montelukast sodium. Post-

Protocol No.: xx/xx/xxx   **Status: Final; Version: 1.0**
This document contains confidential information which is the property of (Name of The Sponsor). It is intended for your internal use only. Do not copy, disclose, or circulate externally without written authorization.
**Date: ....

marketing reports with montelukast sodium use include agitation, aggressive behavior or hostility, anxiousness, depression, disorientation, disturbance in attention, dream abnormalities, hallucinations, insomnia, irritability, memory impairment, restlessness, somnambulism, suicidal thinking and behavior (including suicide), and tremor.

Eosinophilic Conditions: Patients with asthma on therapy with montelukast sodium may present with systemic eosinophilia, sometimes presenting with clinical features of vasculitis consistent with Churg-Strauss syndrome. These events have been sometimes associated with the reduction of oral corticosteroid therapy. Physicians should be alert to eosinophilia, vasculitic rash, worsening pulmonary symptoms, cardiac complications, and/or neuropathy presenting in their patients.

Dosage and Administration

Asthma: Montelukast sodium should be taken once daily in the evening. The following doses are recommended:

> ➤ For adults and adolescents 15 yrs of age and older: one 10 mg dose
> ➤ For pediatric patients 6 to 14 yrs of age: one 5 mg dose
> ➤ For pediatric patients 2 to 5 yrs of age: one 4 mg dose

Exercise-Induced Bronchoconstriction (EIB): For prevention of EIB, a single dose of montelukast should be taken at least 2 hrs before exercise. An additional dose of montelukast should not be taken within 24 hrs of a previous dose. Patients already taking montelukast sodium daily for another indication (including chronic asthma) should not take an additional dose to prevent EIB. Safety and effectiveness in patients younger than 6 yrs of age have not been established. Daily administration of montelukast sodium for the chronic treatment of asthma has not been established to prevent acute episodes of EIB.

Allergic Rhinitis: For allergic rhinitis, montelukast sodium should be taken once daily. Efficacy was demonstrated for seasonal allergic rhinitis when montelukast was administered in the morning or the evening without regard to time of food ingestion. The time of administration may be individualized to suit patient needs. The following doses for the treatment of symptoms of seasonal allergic rhinitis are recommended:

> ➤ For adults and adolescents 15 yrs of age and older: one 10 mg dose
> ➤ For pediatric patients 6 to 14 yrs of age: one 5 mg dose.
> ➤ For pediatric patients 2 to 5 yrs of age: one 4 mg dose.

Protocol No.: xx/xx/xxx   **Status: Final; Version: 1.0**
This document contains confidential information which is the property of (Name of The Sponsor). It is intended for your internal use only. Do not copy, disclose, or circulate externally without written authorization.
Date: ....

The following doses for the treatment of symptoms of perennial allergic rhinitis are recommended:

- ➢ For adults and adolescents 15 yrs of age and older: one 10 mg dose
- ➢ For pediatric patients 6 to 14 yrs of age: one 5 mg dose
- ➢ For pediatric patients 2 to 5 yrs of age: one 4 mg dose

Asthma and Allergic Rhinitis: Patients with both asthma and allergic rhinitis should take only one montelukast sodium dose daily in the evening.

Storage: Tablets should be stored at 15°C-30°C

2.0   Objective

The objective of this study is to compare the oral bioavailability of montelukast orally disintegrating strip 10 mg (each orally disintegrating strip containing montelukast sodium IP equivalent to montelukast 10 mg) manufactured by (name of the sponsor) with marketed samples of spiromont 10 mg orally disintegrating strip (each orally disintegrating strip containing montelukast sodium IP equivalent to montelukast 10 mg) manufactured by (name of the company) in 16+2 or 24+2 healthy, adult, human, male subjects under fasting conditions.

3.0   Study Design

This is a randomized, open label, two treatments, two periods, single dose, crossover bioequivalence study under fasting conditions.

3.1   Sample Size Estimation

Formal sample size estimation was not done for this study 16+2 or 24+2 Healthy; adult, human, male subjects will be enrolled in the study to meet the study objective.

3.2   Treatments

Test Drug [A2]:	Montelukast orally disintegrating strip 10 mg (each orally disintegrating strip containing Montelukast Sodium IP equivalent to Montelukast 10 mg) manufactured by the sponsor
Reference Drug [A1]:	Spiromont 10 mg orally disintegrating strip (each orally disintegrating strip containing Montelukast Sodium IP equivalent to Montelukast 10 mg) manufactured by (name of the company)

3.3   Number of Subjects

16+2 or 24+2 healthy, adult, human, male subjects will be enrolled in the study to meet the study objective.

3.4   Blood Samples

In each of the study period, 11 blood samples will be collected in 5 mL K_2EDTA vacutainers via an indwelling catheter placed in one of the forearm vein. Heparin-lock technique will be used to prevent clotting of blood in the indwelling catheter. Before each blood sample is drawn through catheter, 0.5 mL of blood will be discarded so as to purge the heparinised blood sample in the catheter. Blood samples will also be collected by direct venipuncture during ambulatory blood sampling visit aswell as wherever necessary for any practical reason. The pre-dose blood sample will be collected within a period of 1 hr prior to the drug administration. The post-dose blood samples will be collected at 0.5, 1.0, 2.0, 2.5, 3.0, 4.0, 6.0, 8.0, 12.0 and 24.0 hrs. The total volume of blood drawn including the volume necessary for the laboratory tests [screening & safety sample], PK analysis and the volume of blood discarded before each blood draw will be about 129 mL per subject for the entire study.

Amount of blood drawn for analysis [11 samples × 5mL each× 2 period]	110 mL
Volume of blood discarded before sampling [9 samples× 0.5 mL each × 2 period]	9 mL
Amount of blood drawn at the time of screening [including repeat samples, if required]	10 mL
Total volume of blood drawn per subject for the entire study	**129 mL**

3.5   Study Meals

Supervised fast for at least 10.0 hr before dosing will be maintained in each period. On dosing days lunch, snacks and dinner will be served at 4.0, 8.0 and 14.0 hr post dose respectively. Meal plans will be identical for both the periods. Water will be permitted ad libitum except for 1.0 hr before drug administration and until 1.0 hr post-dose.

This document contains confidential information which is the property of (Name of The Sponsor). It is intended for your internal use only. Do not copy, disclose, or circulate externally without written authorization.
Date: ....

Flow Chart of the Study

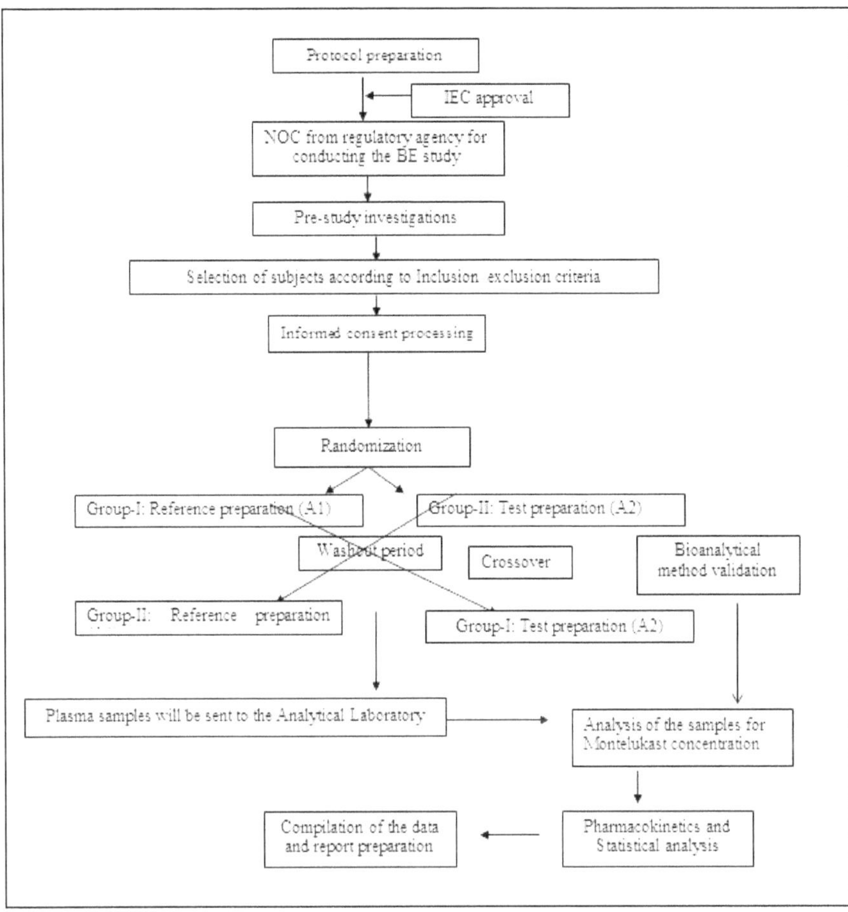

3.6 Housing

Housing from at least 11 hr prior to drug administration until after the 24 hr blood sampling.

3.7 Washout Period

At least 7 days gap between two dosing days will be maintained.

3.8 Vital Signs

Clinical examination and vital signs measurement [blood pressure, pulse rate, respiration rate and oral temperature] will be carried out and recorded

Protocol No.: xx/xx/xxx   **Status: Final; Version: 1.0**
This document contains confidential information which is the property of (Name of The Sponsor). It is intended for your internal use only. Do not copy, disclose, or circulate externally without written authorization.
**Date: ....

at check-in and at check-out. Vital signs [blood pressure and pulse rate] will also be recorded before dosing of investigational products and post dose. Clinical examination and measurement of vital signs may also be carried out at any time during the conduct of the study if the Investigator/Doctor feels necessary. In case of abnormality in pre-dose vital signs, medical opinion will be taken whether to dose the subject or not. During recording of vital sign each subject will be asked about his well-being.

3.9   Analytical Methods

Validated LC-MS/MS method will be used for determination of Montelukast concentration in plasma at Bioanalytical Laboratory of the CRO.

4.0   Subject Selection and Restriction
4.1   Subjects

The study will include 16+2 or 24+2 healthy, adult, human, male subjects, within age of 18-45 yrs, normal BMI [18.5 to 24.99 kg/m^2] and with a minimum weight of 50 kg.

4.2   Subject Screening

Screening for eligibility will be based on inclusion and exclusion criteria. The ICF should be signed by the subject or his/her legally accepted representative before performing any study related assessments on the subject. Once the ICF is signed the subject will undergo complete clinical evaluation. Medical histories and demographic data including initial, sex, age, race, weight [kg], height [cm], BMI [kg/m^2], occupation, alcohol consumption and smoking habits will be recorded.

Laboratory tests to be performed during screening visit:

- **Haematology**
  - Haemoglobin
  - WBC Count
  - Neutrophils
  - Lymphocytes
  - Monocytes
  - Eosinophils
  - Basophils

- **Serum Chemistry**
  - Cholesterol
  - Random Blood Sugar
  - Blood urea &Creatinine
  - Sodium, potassium
  - Uric acid

- LFT
  - ✓ Alk phosphatase
  - ✓ SGPT
  - ✓ Total proteins
  - ✓ Albumin, globulin
  - ✓ Total   Direct bilirubin

Protocol No.: xx/xx/xxx   **Status: Final; Version: 1.0**
This document contains confidential information which is the property of (Name of The Sponsor). It is intended for your internal use only. Do not copy, disclose, or circulate externally without written authorization.
Date: ....

Each subject will undergo a complete physical examination and laboratory tests of haematopoietic, hepatic and renal functions as listed below. Only medically healthy adult human subjects with clinically acceptable/clinically not significant laboratory profiles will be enrolled into the study. The screening will be processed before 48 hrs prior to administration of study drug.

4.3 Inclusion Criteria

- Healthy adult human male subjects within the age range of 18 to 45 yrs.

- Weight not less than 50 kg; Normal BMI [18.5 to 24.99 kg/m^2].

- Willingness to provide written Informed Consent to participate in the study.

- Normal blood pressure and heart rate as measured after resting supine for three minutes.

- Free of significant diseases or clinically significant abnormal findings during screening, medical history, physical examination, laboratory evaluations.

- Absence of disease markers of HIV 1 and 2, Hepatitis B and Syphilis.

- No subject should have received any medication [including over-the-counter products] for 14 days preceding the start of the study.

- No history of drug abuse (benzodiazepines and barbiturates) for the last one month and other illicit drugs for the last 6 months.

- To be a non-smoker.

- The volunteer should be able to communicate well with the investigator.

- Availability of subject for the entire study period and willingness to adhere to protocol requirements as evidence by written informed consent.

4.4 Exclusion Criteria

- History or presence of significant cardiovascular, pulmonary, hepatic, renal, hematological, gastro-intestinal, endocrine, immunologic, dermatologic, neurological, psychiatric disease.

- History or presence of significant:

This document contains confidential information which is the property of (Name of The Sponsor). It is intended for your internal use only. Do not copy, disclose, or circulate externally without written authorization.
**Date: ....

- ➢ Alcohol dependence, alcohol abuse or drug abuse during past one year.
- ➢ Asthma, urticaria or other allergic type reactions after taking aspirin or any other drug.
- ➢ Ulceration or history of gastric and / or duodenal ulcer.
- ➢ Jaundice in the past 6 months.

- Bleeding disorder and Maintenance therapy with any drug
- Poor mental development or impaired cerebral function.
- Allergy to the Test drug or any drug chemically similar to the drug or to the excipients of the products under investigation.
- 1 unit or 350 mL blood loss within 56 days prior to start of study.
- Subjects who have participated in another clinical study in the past 3 months prior to commencement of this study.
- Any difficulty in accessibility of forearm veins for cannulation or blood sampling.
- Refuse to abstain from food for at least 10 hrs prior to drug administration and for at least 4 hrs after drug administration in each period.
- Refuse to abstain from fluid for at least 1 hr prior to drug administration and until 1 hr after drug administration.
- Found positive in breath alcohol test on the day of check-in.
- History of difficulty in swallowing tablet.
- Use of enzyme modifying drugs within 30 days prior to receiving the first dose of study medication.
- Hypersensitivity to Montelukast and other related class of drugs.

4.5   Criteria for Subject Withdrawal

Subjects will be free to withdraw at any time without stating any reason. The Investigator may withdraw a subject from the study if:

- The subject suffers from significant intercurrent illness or undergoes surgery during the course of the study.
- The subject experiences adverse event, when withdrawal would be in the best interest of the subjects.
- If the subject requires concomitant medications which may interfere with the pharmacokinetics of study drug.

This document contains confidential information which is the property of (Name of The Sponsor). It is intended for your internal use only. Do not copy, disclose, or circulate externally without written authorization.
Date: ....

- If the Investigator thinks it is necessary to further protect the health of the subject or the integrity of the study.

- If subject vomits at or before the time equivalent to 2 median T_{max} after administration of investigational product.

- The subject fails to comply with the requirements of the protocol.

Any subject discontinuing the trial medication prematurely because of reasons 1 or 5 will be replaced. The final report will include reasons for withdrawals.

4.6 Prohibitions

No subject should have received any medication [including over-the-counter products] for 14 days preceding the study. This prohibition includes vitamins taken as nutritional supplements for non-therapeutic indication as judged by the Investigator/ Doctor. If concomitant medication is required during the time of sample collection or during the washout period between drug administrations, a decision to continue or discontinue the subjects will be made based on the time the medication was administered and its pharmacology and pharmacokinetics by the Investigator.

No subject should have smoked at least 24 hrs before check-in and smoking will be prohibited throughout the study period. No subject should have taken alcoholic beverages at least 48.0 hrs before check-in. No subject should have taken xanthine containing beverages and food or grape fruit juice at least 48.0 hrs before check-in and the same will be prohibited throughout the study period. No strenuous exercises during the whole study period will be permitted.

4.7 Subject Data Identification

The subject will be identified by volunteer/subject ID Number. All the volunteers enrolled into the study will be given subject number serially as per their reporting time in period one which will remain same throughout the study. Data of each subject will be identified either by the subject registration number or subject number.

5.0 Clinical Procedures

5.1 Investigational Product Administration

As per the randomization schedule, single ODS (Orally Disintegrating Strip) of either Test or Reference product will be orally administered to

Protocol No.: xx/xx/xxx   **Status: Final; Version: 1.0**
This document contains confidential information which is the property of (Name of The Sponsor). It is intended for your internal use only. Do not copy, disclose, or circulate externally without written authorization.
Date: ....

each subject in each period in sitting posture after an overnight fast of at least 10 hr. Both the test product and reference product will be given to the volunteers without water initially and after complete disintegration of the strip, 240 ml of water will be provided. Compliance for the dosing will be assessed by checking the oral cavity immediately after dosing. Subjects will remain in upright position [sitting or ambulatory] for 2.0 hr post-dose in each period except when clinically indicated to change the posture. The subjects will receive a standardized meal only after 4.0 hr post-dose. Water will be permitted *ad libitum* except for 1.0 hr before and until 1.0 hr post-dose.

5.2   Blood Sample Handling

Blood samples will be collected in 5 mL K_2EDTA vacutainers at specified time. Any blood draws after the window period of 2 min will be noted as a sampling time point deviation except pre-dose blood sample. Blood samples will be drawn via an indwelling catheter using heparin-lock technique or by direct venipuncture. Before each in-house blood draw, 0.5 mL of blood will be discarded so as to purge heparinised blood in the catheter. Immediately after collection of blood, the sample will be kept in ice bath. All the blood samples for a particular sample time point will be centrifuged under refrigeration [at 3500 rpm and 4°C for 10 min]. The time interval between sample collection and the start of centrifugation should not exceed more than 45 min. The resulting plasma will be separated and stored in suitably labeled polypropylene tubes at -20 ± 2°C for pending assay.

5.3   Activity Levels

Subjects will remain upright [sitting or ambulatory] for the first 2.0 hr post-dose in both the study periods. However, should medical events occur at any time, subject may be placed in an appropriate position. Subjects will be monitored throughout confinement for adverse events. No strenuous exercises will be permitted.

5.4   Adverse Event Monitoring and Reporting

The Principal Investigator will monitor safety data throughout the course of the study. A qualified medical officer experienced in conducting bioequivalence study will be available during housing in the clinical center.

This document contains confidential information which is the property of (Name of The Sponsor). It is intended for your internal use only. Do not copy, disclose, or circulate externally without written authorization.
Date: ....

Subjects will be monitored throughout the study period for occurrence of adverse events. A nearby nursing home attached with the CRO capable of handling emergency situations will be informed about the study. In case of adverse event, if required, the physicians attached to the hospital will treat adverse events as appropriate, either at the study center or with the Hospital. Subjects experiencing adverse events will be followed up until resolution of adverse event. Subjects who at least receive one dose of the study medication will be included in the safety analysis.

5.5   Adverse Events

The following definitions will be used in assessment and recording of an adverse event:

Adverse event [AE]: An AE is any untoward medical occurrence in a patient or clinical investigation subject administered a pharmaceutical product and that does not necessarily have a causal relationship with this treatment. An AE can therefore be any unfavorable and unintended sign (including an abnormal laboratory finding), symptom, or disease temporally associated with the use of a medicinal (investigational) product, whether or not related to the medicinal (investigational) product.

Adverse drug reaction [ADR]: All noxious and unintended responses to a medical product related to any dose should be considered an adverse drug reaction.

The expectedness of an ADR to the study medication should be graded as follows:

Expected drug reaction: An adverse reaction, the nature or severity of which is consistent with applicable product labeling (e.g. the investigator brochure for an approved experimental drug; the data sheet (or package insert) for a marketed product).

Unexpected adverse drug reaction: An adverse reaction, the nature or severity of which is not consistent with applicable product labeling (e.g. the investigator brochure for an approved experimental drug; the data sheet (or package insert) for a marketed product).

Serious adverse event: A serious adverse event or reaction is an untoward medical occurrence that at any dose:

- Results in death;

Protocol No.: xx/xx/xxx   **Status: Final; Version: 1.0**
This document contains confidential information which is the property of (Name of The Sponsor). It is intended for your internal use only. Do not copy, disclose, or circulate externally without written authorization.
Date: ....

- Is life-threatening;

- Requires in-patient hospitalization or prolongation of existing hospitalization;

- Results in persistent or significant disability/incapacity;

- Leads to any congenital anomaly;

- Necessitates medical or surgical intervention to preclude permanent impairment of a body function or permanent damage to body structure.

The term "life-threatening" in the definition of "serious" refers to an event in which the patient was at risk of death due to the adverse event at severity it occurred; it does not refer to an event which might have caused death if it occurred in more severe form. Examples of such events are intensive treatment in an emergency room or at home for allergic bronchospasm; blood dispraises or convulsions that do not result in hospitalization; or development of drug dependency or drug abuse. All serious adverse events will be reported within 7 working days to the IEC/IRB (Ethics Review Committee) approving the study. Occurrence of any Serious Adverse Event [SAE] needs to be notified by the Investigator to the sponsor immediately [within 24 hr of becoming aware of the occurrence of the event]. As soon as new information about the SAE becomes known the Investigator has to forward it without delay to the sponsor.

Non-serious adverse event: All AEs which are not considered to be serious whether expected or not should be described as 'non-serious' for the purposes of reporting. All adverse events, unless specified, refer to non-serious adverse events. The causal relationship of an AE to the study medication/device should be graded as follows:

None: The AE is definitely not associated with the study medication/device administered.

Unlikely/Remote: The temporal association is such that the study medication/device is not likely to have had an association with observed AE.

Possible: This causal relationship is assigned when the AE: (a) follows a reasonable temporal sequence from medication/device administration but: (b) could have been produced by the study subject's clinical state or other modes of therapy administered to the study subject.

Protocol No.: xx/xx/xxx   **Status: Final; Version: 1.0**
This document contains confidential information which is the property of (Name of The Sponsor). It is intended for your internal use only. Do not copy, disclose, or circulate externally without written authorization.
Date: ....

Probable: This causal relationship is assigned when the AE: (a) follows a reasonable temporal sequence from medication/device administration; (b) abates upon discontinuation of the treatment; (c) cannot be reasonably explained by known characteristics of the study subject's clinical state.

Highly probable: This causal relationship is assigned when the AE: (a) follows a reasonable temporal sequence from medication/device administration; (b) abates upon discontinuation of the treatment; and (c) is confirmed by reappearance of the AE on repeat exposure (rechallenge).

In assessable: (a) more data for proper assessment needed; cannot be judged because information is insufficient or contradictory at the time of assessment; (b) additional details under examination; (c) Details cannot be supplemented or verified.

Severity (intensity) of AE should be assessed according to following definitions:

Mild: The AE is transient, requires no treatment, and does not interfere with the study subject's daily activities.

Moderate: The AE introduces a low level of inconvenience or concern to the study subject and may interfere with daily activities, but is usually ameliorated by simple therapeutic measures.

Severe: The AE interrupts the study subject's usual daily activity and requires systematic therapy or other treatment.

Subjects will be monitored throughout confinement for adverse events. A doctor will be on the premises during the drug administration in each period and until the end of the housing period. Clinical examination and vital signs [blood pressure, pulse rate and oral temperature] will be carried out and recorded at each check-in and at check-out. Vital signs [blood pressure and pulse rate] will also be recorded before dosing of investigational products and post-dose. Clinical examination and measurement of vital signs may also be carried out at any time during the conduct of the study if the Investigator/Doctor feels it necessary. In case of abnormality in pre-dose vital signs, medical opinion will be taken whether to dose the subject or not. During recording of vital signs each subject will be asked about his well-being. At the end of clinical stay an exit interview will be conducted during check-out.

Any subject who develops any adverse event or clinically significant abnormal laboratory test values will be evaluated, and will be treated and /or followed up until the symptoms or values return to normal or acceptable

Protocol No.: xx/xx/xxx   **Status: Final; Version: 1.0**
This document contains confidential information which is the property of (Name of The Sponsor). It is intended for your internal use only. Do not copy, disclose, or circulate externally without written authorization.
Date: ....

levels, as judged by the Investigator /Doctor. A doctor, either at nearby hospital's emergency room, will be available to administer treatment for any serious adverse event.

6.0   Data Analysis

6.1   Pharmacokinetic Analysis

Pharmacokinetic parameters for Montelukast will be calculated using 'SAS version 9.1.3/WinNonlin^{TM} Enterprise V:5.3,' as follows:

AUC_{0-t}	The area under the plasma concentration versus time curve, from time 0 to the last measurable concentration, as calculated by the linear trapezoidal method.
$AUC_{0-\infty}$	The area under the plasma concentration versus time curve from time 0 to infinity. $AUC_{0-\infty}$ is calculated as the sum of the AUC_{0-t} and the ratio of the last measurable plasma concentration to the elimination rate constant.
C_{max}	Maximum measured plasma concentration over the time span specified
T_{max}	Time of the maximum measured plasma concentration. If the maximum value occurs at more than one time point, T_{max} is defined as the first time point with this value.
$t_{1/2}$	The elimination or terminal half-life will be calculated as $0.693/K_{el}$, where K_{el} = elimination rate constant estimated from the slope of terminal linear portion of the plasma concentration time curve
K_{el}	Elimination rate constant estimated from the slope of terminal linear portion of the plasma concentration-time curve

Pharmacokinetic analysis will be performed for all the subjects who complete both the periods of the study. If necessary, an unequal number of subjects per sequence will be used for pharmacokinetic analysis.

No value of K_{el}, $AUC_{0-\infty}$ or $t_{1/2}$ will be reported for cases that do not exhibit a terminal log-linear phase in the concentration versus time profile.

6.2   Statistical Analysis

Statistical analyses will be performed for pharmacokinetic parameters of Test and Reference formulation using the SAS version 9.1.3/ WinNonlin (Version 5.3) [Pharsight Corporation, USA]. Statistical analysis will be done for all the subjects who complete all the periods of the study.

6.3   Summary Statistics

Arithmetic mean, standard deviation, minimum, maximum, median, range, percentage co-efficient of variation (%CV), standard error and geometric

Protocol No.: xx/xx/xxx   **Status: Final; Version: 1.0**
This document contains confidential information which is the property of (Name of The Sponsor). It is intended for your internal use only. Do not copy, disclose, or circulate externally without written authorization.
Date: ....

mean will be calculated for the parameters listed in section 6.1 for both Test and Reference formulations.

6.4   Analysis of Variance

The log-transformed pharmacokinetic parameters [C_{max}, AUC_{0-t} & $AUC_{0-\infty}$] will be analyzed using a Mixed Effects ANOVA Model using Type III sum of squares with the main effects of Treatment, Period and Sequence as Fixed Effects and Subjects nested within Sequence as Random Effect. A separate ANOVA model will be used to analyze each of the parameters. The sequence effect will be tested at 0.10 level of significance using the subjects nested within sequence mean square as the error term, and all other main effects will be tested at the 0.05 level of significance using the residual error (mean square error) from the ANOVA model as the error term. Each analysis of variance will include calculation of least-square mean for Test and Reference formulations, the difference between the least-square means and the standard error associated with the difference of means. The above analyses will be done using the appropriate WinNonlin software.

6.5   Ratio Analysis and 90% Confidence Intervals

Ratio and 90% Confidence Interval for the Test/Reference ratio will be calculated using least square mean differences and standard error of difference of means for Test and Reference formulations obtained from ANOVA for log-transformed C_{max}, AUC_{0-t} and $AUC_{0-\infty}$. The Confidence Intervals will be expressed as percentage.

6.6   Intra-subject and Inter-subject Variability

Intra-subject variability and inter-subject variability will be calculated using residual error (mean square error) and mean sum of squares due to subject nested within the sequence obtained from ANOVA for log-transformed C_{max}, AUC_{0-t} and $AUC_{0-\infty}$.

6.7   Bioequivalence Criteria

The calculated 90% Confidence Interval for Montelukast should fall within 80 to 125% for the Test / Reference ratios for AUC_{0-t}, $AUC_{0-\infty}$ and C_{max} to conclude bioequivalence.

Protocol No.: xx/xx/xxx   **Status: Final; Version: 1.0**
This document contains confidential information which is the property of (Name of The Sponsor). It is intended for your internal use only. Do not copy, disclose, or circulate externally without written authorization.
Date: ....

7.0   Clinical Supplies

The Sponsor will supply sufficient quantities of the study formulations to allow completion of this study. The drug products will be received by the Investigator/Pharmacist or a suitable designate from the Human Pharmacology Unit department along with the Certificate of Analysis [COA]. Reference products will be supplied in the manufacturer's original packing material and the test products will be supplied in an appropriate package deemed to maintain the integrity of the products. Dispensing would be done by CRO on each check-in day. Records will be made of the receipt, dispensing and the unused clinical supplies to provide a complete accountability of the supplied investigational product. The clinical supplies will be stored at prescribed storage conditions in a secured facility accessible only to the Investigator or authorized personnel. The batch numbers, expiry dates and physical description of investigational products will also be included in the study report. Remaining quantity of samples will be stored for minimum of 5 yrs after the completion of the study or as intimated by the Sponsor based on the regulatory requirements.

7.1   Assignment to Treatment Sequences

The order of receiving the Test and Reference products for each subject during all periods of the study will be determined according to a computer generated randomization schedule. The Investigator and Pharmacist will be accountable for ensuring compliance to randomization schedule.

7.2   Assessment of Treatment Compliance

Compliance will be assessed by conducting a mouth check by a trained study personnel after dosing in each period and by measurement of Montelukast concentration in plasma [during the analytical phase of the study].

8.0   Ethical Considerations

8.1   Basic Principles

This research will be carried out in accordance with the clinical research guidelines established by the basic principles and the principles enunciated in The Declaration of Helsinki, Ethical Principles for Medical Research Involving Human Subjects [59th WMA General Assembly, Seoul, October 2008] and as per ICMR and Indian GCP guidelines.

8.2   Independent Ethics Committee

This protocol, Informed Consent Form along with protocol appendices will be reviewed by Independent Bioethics Committee. The study subjects will be dosed only after the IEC has approved the protocol, Informed Consent Form along with protocol appendices or a modification thereof, except for medical screening of volunteers to record their health status after their consent for screening. IEC consultants operate in compliance with ICH-GCP, ICMR guidelines, Guidelines for Clinical Trials– CDCSO (India) and Schedule Y of Drugs & Cosmetics Act & Rules.

8.3   Informed Consent

Prior to enrollment into the study, the Investigator/designated person will inform the volunteer about purpose of the study, the procedures to be carried out, the potential hazards and rights of the volunteer in a language that the subject comprehends. Ample time and opportunity will be provided to volunteer for deciding to or not to participate in the study. The subjects will be required to read and sign the consent form summarizing the discussion prior to enrollment. A copy of the Informed Consent Form will be given to the subject, which describes the study procedures and potential hazards in non-technical terms in conformity with regulatory requirements. By signing the consent form, the subject attests that the information in the consent form and any other written information was accurately explained to and apparently understood by the subject and that the Informed Consent was given freely by the subject.

In case of illiterate volunteers, a Legally Acceptable Representative / Impartial Witness will be present at the times of providing information and obtaining consent from the volunteer. The non-dominant hand thumb impression of volunteer will be obtained on all pages of the Informed Consent Form. Legally Acceptable Representative /Witness will be asked to sign and date the appropriate section of Informed Consent Form.

8.4   Confidentiality

All data generated from the study will be regarded as confidential. The monitor(s), the auditor(s), the IRB/IEC, and the regulatory authority(ies) will be granted direct access to the subject's original medical records for verification of study procedures and/or data, without violating the confidentiality of the subject, to the extent permitted by the applicable laws and regulations and that, by signing a written Informed Consent Form, the subject or the subject's legally acceptable representative will be authorizing such access.The records identifying the subject will be kept confidential and, to the extent permitted by the applicable laws and/or regulations, will not be made publicly available. If the results of the trial are published, the subject's identity will remain confidential. No publication or dissemination of the data will be permitted without prior written agreement with the Sponsor.

8.5   Compensation, Insurance and Indemnity

Subjects must understand that the study will be performed for research purposes only and that no therapeutic benefit may be expected as a consequence of their involvement. In addition, each subject must understand that participation in the study may involve risks which are currently unforeseeable. If any of the volunteers subjected to physical injury or death because of study drug the **Sponsor** will provide complete medical assistance as well as compensation for the injury or death, as per The Government of India, Gazette Notification No. GSR 53 (E) dated 30.01.2013 and amended vide GSR 889 (E) dated 12.12.2014.

8.6   Payment to Subjects

Payment will be made to subjects for the time and inconvenience of the study at a level to be decided by the Investigator. The precise level of payment will be subject as per the CDSCO (India), GSR 53 (E) dated 30.01.2013 and amended vide GSR 889 (E) dated 12.12.2014. Subjects who fail to complete the study will be paid at the discretion of the Investigator. Those subjects who are withdrawn by the Investigator after suffering an adverse reaction to the study medication will receive full payment. Those subjects who voluntarily withdraw will receive proportionate payment.

8.7   Termination of the Study

The Sponsor reserves the right to terminate the study at any time. Reasons for this termination will be provided to the subjects. The Principal Investigator reserves the right to discontinue the study for safety reasons at any time.

9.0   Analytical Procedures

Validated LC-MS/MS method will be employeed for determination of

Montelukast concerntration in plasma samples. During the analysis, standard and quality control samples will be distributed throughout each batch of study samples analyzed. The analyst will not have access to the randomization scheme. The method validation involve the essential parameters such as selectivity, sensitivity, precision, accuracy, recovery, freeze-thaw stability, long term stability, short term stability and matrix effect. All concentration values below the limit of quantification will be set to zero for all pharmacokinetic and statistical evaluation. Any missing samples will be reported as 'M' and for any unreportable concentration values will be reported as 'NR' and will not be included for pharmacokinetic or statistical analysis.

Plasma samples of the subjects who completed the study will be analyzed. Subjects who are withdrawn from the study due to an adverse event related to study drug will also be assayed. Their concentration data will be provided in separate table and will not be included in pharmacokinetic and statistical analysis.

Analysis of Plasma Samples

Standard solutions: Separate solutions containing 1 mg/ml of analytes and I.S. should be prepared using mobile phase respectively. These solutions will be further diluted suitably with the mobile phase to obtain a stock solution of 1 µg/ml. The stock solutions prepared for the drugs will be diluted further to obtain eight working solutions for calibration standards. All solutions must be stored at 2–8°C.

Calibration curves: An eight point standard calibration solutions of analyte(s) should be prepared by spiking appropriate amounts of analyte(s) and IS in human plasma to yield final concentrations. Three quality control (QC) samples will be prepared at three concentration levels of analyte. Calibration curves will be plotted with peak area ratio of drug and IS on Y- axis and concentration on X- axis.

Sample preparation and extraction: Liquid-liquid extraction procedure should be used for the extraction of the drug from the plasma. Calibration standards, quality control samples will be treated with 5 ml of organic solvent. 100 µl of internal standard be added with each 1 ml plasma sample and vortex mixed for 10 min followed by centrifugation for another 10 min. The organic layer containing the analyte(s) will be separated, transferred to a separate test tube and evaporated to dryness under a stream of N_2 at 40°C. The residue obtained on drying will be reconstituted with the 250 µl of mobile phase/diluent. The reconstituted sample will be manually with the

Protocol No.: xx/xx/xxx   **Status: Final; Version: 1.0**
This document contains confidential information which is the property of (Name of The Sponsor). It is intended for your internal use only. Do not copy, disclose, or circulate externally without written authorization.
Date: ....

micro liter syringe into the injector with fixed volume loop and will be injected into the liquid chromatography system.

10.0 Treatment of Time Point Deviation

Time deviation for any subject at any time point will be taken care, while calculation of pharmacokinetic parameters.

11.0 Procedure for Reporting any Deviation(S) from the Original Statistical Plan

The deviations from planned analysis of protocol will be documented in the final report as a protocol deviation.

12.0 Study Report and Documents

The final report will be written according to the ICH guidelines (Guideline for Structure and Content of Clinical Study Reports). The report will contain data regarding the analytical methodology and the chromatograms of at least 20% of the serially selected subjects, the pharmacokinetic and statistical analysis data, and a clinical report.

13.0 Supplementary Documentation

A sample Informed Consent Form, IEC approval of the study, COA of Test and Reference products, randomization schedule, and other required documents will be filed with the final report.

14.0 Archives

All raw data generated in connection with this study, together with the original copy of the final report, will be retained for 5 years in the archives of the CRO.

15.0 Direct Access to Source Data/Documents

Direct access to source data/documents will be permitted to study-related monitoring, audits, IEC review and regulatory inspection(s).

16.0 Quality Control and Quality Assurance

The raw data generated during the course of the study as well as reports will undergo quality assurance by the Quality Assurance personnel audit for conformance to this protocol and all the governing SOPs. The final

Protocol No.: xx/xx/xxx   **Status: Final; Version: 1.0**
This document contains confidential information which is the property of (Name of The Sponsor). It is intended for your internal use only. Do not copy, disclose, or circulate externally without written authorization.
Date: ....

report will contain a Quality Assurance Statement duly signed by the Quality Assurance personnel. The Sponsor may also perform audit for the study.

17.0 Publication

The Investigator will not publish the data collected during the course of this study in any form, except with the written permission of the Sponsor. Any data published will not reveal the identity of any study subjects, and confidentiality will be maintained. Any member of the research team including those employed by the Sponsor who makes a real contribution to the preparation of publications may be included amongst the authors of the paper(s) prepared.

18.0 Changes in Protocol

The Investigator will not implement any changes to the approved protocol without agreement from the Sponsor and prior review and documented approval from the IEC of an amendment, except where necessary to eliminate an immediate hazard(s) to trial subjects, or when the change(s) involves only logistical or administrative aspects of the trial.

The following definitions & details will be used while assessment & recording of protocol deviations/violation:

Protocol Deviation: Any alteration/modification to the IEC-approved protocol. The protocol includes the detailed protocol, protocol summary, consent form, recruitment materials, questionnaires, and any other information relating to the research study. Protocol deviation can also be known as planned protocol deviation because it protocol deviation will be approved by IEC prior to its implementation.

Major Deviation: A major protocol deviation is a deviation that has an impact on subject safety, may substantially alter risks to subjects, may have an effect on the integrity of the study data, or may affect the subject's willingness to participate in the study.

Minor Deviation: A minor protocol deviation is one that does not impact subject safety, compromise the integrity of the study data, or affect the subject's willingness to participate in the study.

The Protocol deviations will be recorded in "Protocol Amendment Form" and same will be reported in final study report.

Protocol No.: xx/xx/xxx   **Status: Final; Version: 1.0**

This document contains confidential information which is the property of (Name of The Sponsor). It is intended for your internal use only. Do not copy, disclose, or circulate externally without written authorization.

Date: ....

Protocol Violation: Any protocol deviation that is not approved by the IEC prior to its initiation or implementation. Protocol Violation is also known as unplanned protocol deviation.

Major Violation: A major protocol violation is a deviation that has an impact on subject safety, may substantially alter risks to subjects, may have an effect on the integrity of the study data, or may affect the subject's willingness to participate in the study.

Minor Violation: A minor protocol violation is one that does not impact subject safety, compromise the integrity of the study data, or affect the subject's willingness to participate in the study.

The Protocol violations will be recorded in "Protocol Violation Form" and same will be reported in final study report.

19.0 References

- Miyako Kishimoto, Montelukast: a DPP-4 inhibitor for the treatment of type 2 diabetes, Diabetes, Metabolic Syndrome and Obesity: Targets and Therapy 2013:6 187–195.

- Atef Halabi, Haidar Maatouk, Karl Ernst Siegler, Nadja Faisst, Volkmar Lufft, and Norbert Klause, Pharmacokinetics of Montelukast in Subjects With Renal Impairment; Clinical Pharmacology in Drug Development 2(3) 246–254.

- Yoshinobu Nakamaru, Yoshiharu Hayashi, Ruriko Ikegawa, Shuji Kinoshita4, Begonya Perez Madera,Dave Gunput, Atsuhiro Kawaguchi, Martin Davies, Stuart Mair, Hiroshi Yamazaki, Toshiyuki Kume, and Masayuki Suzuki, Metabolism and disposition of the dipeptidyl peptidase IV inhibitor Montelukast in humans, Xenobiotica, 2014; 44(3): 242–253.

- Yoshinobu Nakamaru; Yoshiharu Hayashi, Mana Sekine; Shuji Kinoshita; Jeff Thompson, Atsuhiro Kawaguchi, Martin Davies, Horst Ju¨rgen Heuer, Hiroshi Yamazaki, and Kei Akimoto, Effect of Ketoconazole on the Pharmacokinetics of the Dipeptidyl Peptidase-4 inhibitor montelukast: An Open-Label Study in Healthy White Subjects in Germany. Clinical Therapeutics, 2014.

- Yoshinobu Nakamaru, Yoshiharu Hayashi, MartinDavies, Horst Ju¨rgen Heuer, Noriko Hisanaga, and Kei Akimoto, Investigation of Potential Pharmacokinetic Interactions Between Montelukast and Metformin in Steady-State Conditions in Healthy Adults. Clinical Therapeutics, 2015.

Protocol No.: xx/xx/xxx   **Status: Final; Version: 1.0**

This document contains confidential information which is the property of (Name of The Sponsor). It is intended for your internal use only. Do not copy, disclose, or circulate externally without written authorization.

Date: ....

- Raja Haranadha Babu Chunduri and Gowri Sankar Dannana., Development and validation of LC-MS/MS method for quantification of Montelukast in human plasma and its application to a pharmacokinetic study. World journal of pharmacy and pharmaceutical sciences. Volume 5, Issue 5, 838-850.

20.0 List of Appendices

- **Appendix I**   Declaration of Helsinki
- **Appendix II**   Informed Consent Form, Subject Information Sheet (English & Bengali)
- **Appendix III**   Informed Consent Form [Bengali]
- **Appendix IV**   Schedule of study event
- **Appendix V**   Case Record Form
- **Appendix VI**   Table of Study Diet
- **Appendix VII**   Investigator's undertaking
- **Appendix VIII**   Serious adverse event form
- **Appendix IX**   Utilization Breakup

Protocol No.: xx/xx/xxx   **Status: Final; Version: 1.0**
This document contains confidential information which is the property of (Name of The Sponsor). It is intended for your internal use only. Do not copy, disclose, or circulate externally without written authorization.
Date: ....

Appendix-I

WORLD MEDICAL ASSOCIATION DECLARATION OF HELSINKI

Ethical Principles for Medical Research Involving Human Subjects

Adopted by the 18th WMA General Assembly, Helsinki, Finland, June 1964,
and amended by the:

29th WMA General Assembly, Tokyo, Japan, October 1975

35th WMA General Assembly, Venice, Italy, October 1983

41st WMA General Assembly, Hong Kong, September 1989

48th WMA General Assembly, Somerset West, Republic of South Africa, October 1996

52nd WMA General Assembly, Edinburgh, Scotland, October 2000

53rd WMA General Assembly, Washington 2002 (Note of Clarification on
paragraph 29 added)

55th WMA General Assembly, Tokyo 2004 (Note of Clarification on Paragraph 30 added)

59th WMA General Assembly, Seoul, October 2008

A. INTRODUCTION

1. The World Medical Association (WMA) has developed the Declaration of Helsinki as a statement of ethical principles for medical research involving human subjects, including research on identifiable human material and data.

   The Declaration is intended to be read as a whole and each of its constituent paragraphs should not be applied without consideration of all other relevant paragraphs.

2. Although the Declaration is addressed primarily to physicians, the WMA encourages other participants in medical research involving human subjects to adopt these principles.

3. It is the duty of the physician to promote and safeguard the health of patients, including those who are involved in medical research. The physician's knowledge and conscience are dedicated to the fulfillment of this duty.

4. The Declaration of Geneva of the WMA binds the physician with the words, "The health of my patient will be my first consideration," and the International Code of Medical Ethics declares that, "A physician shall act in the patient's best interest when providing medical care".

Protocol No.: xx/xx/xxx   **Status: Final; Version: 1.0**
This document contains confidential information which is the property of (Name of The Sponsor). It is intended for your internal use only. Do not copy, disclose, or circulate externally without written authorization.
Date: ....

5. Medical progress is based on research that ultimately must include studies involving human subjects. Populations that are underrepresented in medical research should be provided appropriate access to participation in research.

6. In medical research involving human subjects, the well-being of the individual research subject must take precedence over all other interests.

7. The primary purpose of medical research involving human subjects is to understand the causes, development and effects of diseases and improve preventive, diagnostic and therapeutic interventions (methods, procedures and treatments). Even the best current interventions must be evaluated continually through research for their safety, effectiveness, efficiency, accessibility and quality.

8. In medical practice and in medical research, most interventions involve risks and burdens.

9. Medical research is subject to ethical standards that promote respect for all human subjects and protect their health and rights. Some research populations are particularly vulnerable and need special protection. These include those who cannot give or refuse consent for themselves and those who may be vulnerable to coercion or undue influence.

10. Physicians should consider the ethical, legal and regulatory norms and standards for research involving human subjects in their own countries as well as applicable international norms and standards. No national or international ethical, legal or regulatory requirement should reduce or eliminate any of the protections for research subjects set forth in this Declaration.

B. PRINCIPLES FOR ALL MEDICAL RESEARCH

11. It is the duty of physicians who participate in medical research to protect the life, health, dignity, integrity, right to self-determination, privacy, and confidentiality of personal information of research subjects.

12. Medical research involving human subjects must conform to generally accepted scientific principles, be based on a thorough knowledge of the scientific literature, other relevant sources of information, and adequate laboratory and, as appropriate, animal

Protocol No.: xx/xx/xxx   **Status: Final; Version: 1.0**
This document contains confidential information which is the property of (Name of The Sponsor). It is intended for your internal use only. Do not copy, disclose, or circulate externally without written authorization.
Date: ....

experimentation. The welfare of animals used for research must be respected.

13. Appropriate caution must be exercised in the conduct of medical research that may harm the environment.

14. The design and performance of each research study involving human subjects must be clearly described in a research protocol. The protocol should contain a statement of the ethical considerations involved and should indicate how the principles in this Declaration have been addressed. The protocol should include information regarding funding, sponsors, institutional affiliations, other potential conflicts of interest, incentives for subjects and provisions for treating and/or compensating subjects who are harmed as a consequence of participation in the research study. The protocol should describe arrangements for post-study access by study subjects to interventions identified as beneficial in the study or access to other appropriate care or benefits.

15. The research protocol must be submitted for consideration, comment, guidance and approval to a research ethics committee before the study begins. This committee must be independent of the researcher, the sponsor and any other undue influence. It must take into consideration the laws and regulations of the country or countries in which the research is to be performed as well as applicable international norms and standards but these must not be allowed to reduce or eliminate any of the protections for research subjects set forth in this Declaration. The committee must have the right to monitor ongoing studies. The researcher must provide monitoring information to the committee, especially information about any serious adverse events. No change to the protocol may be made without consideration and approval by the committee.

16. Medical research involving human subjects must be conducted only by individuals with the appropriate scientific training and qualifications. Research on patients or healthy volunteers requires the supervision of a competent and appropriately qualified physician or other health care professional. The responsibility for the protection of research subjects must always rest with the physician or other health care professional and never the research subjects, even though they have given consent.

17. Medical research involving a disadvantaged or vulnerable population or community is only justified if the research is responsive to the health needs and priorities of this population or community and if there is a reasonable likelihood that this population or community stands to benefit from the results of the research.

18. Every medical research study involving human subjects must be preceded by careful assessment of predictable risks and burdens to the individuals and communities involved in the research in comparison with foreseeable benefits to them and to other individuals or communities affected by the condition under investigation.

19. Every clinical trial must be registered in a publicly accessible database before recruitment of the first subject.

20. Physicians may not participate in a research study involving human subjects unless they are confident that the risks involved have been adequately assessed and can be satisfactorily managed. Physicians must immediately stop a study when the risks are found to outweigh the potential benefits or when there is conclusive proof of positive and beneficial results.

21. Medical research involving human subjects may only be conducted if the importance of the objective outweighs the inherent risks and burdens to the research subjects.

22. Participation by competent individuals as subjects in medical research must be voluntary. Although it may be appropriate to consult family members or community leaders, no competent individual may be enrolled in a research study unless he or she freely agrees.

23. Every precaution must be taken to protect the privacy of research subjects and the confidentiality of their personal information and to minimize the impact of the study on their physical, mental and social integrity.

24. In medical research involving competent human subjects, each potential subject must be adequately informed of the aims, methods, sources of funding, any possible conflicts of interest, institutional affiliations of the researcher, the anticipated benefits and potential risks of the study and the discomfort it may entail, and any other relevant aspects of the study. The potential subject must be informed

Protocol No.: xx/xx/xxx   **Status: Final; Version: 1.0**
This document contains confidential information which is the property of (Name of The Sponsor). It is intended for your internal use only. Do not copy, disclose, or circulate externally without written authorization.
Date: ....

of the right to refuse to participate in the study or to withdraw consent to participate at any time without reprisal. Special attention should be given to the specific information needs of individual potential subjects as well as to the methods used to deliver the information. After ensuring that the potential subject has understood the information, the physician or another appropriately qualified individual must then seek the potential subject's freely-given informed consent, preferably in writing. If the consent cannot be expressed in writing, the non-written consent must be formally documented and witnessed.

25. For medical research using identifiable human material or data, physicians must normally seek consent for the collection, analysis, storage and/or reuse. There may be situations where consent would be impossible or impractical to obtain for such research or would pose a threat to the validity of the research. In such situations the research may be done only after consideration and approval of a research ethics committee.

26. When seeking informed consent for participation in a research study the physician should be particularly cautious if the potential subject is in a dependent relationship with the physician or may consent under duress. In such situations the informed consent should be sought by an appropriately qualified individual who is completely independent of this relationship.

27. For a potential research subject who is incompetent, the physician must seek informed consent from the legally authorized representative. These individuals must not be included in a research study that has no likelihood of benefit for them unless it is intended to promote the health of the population represented by the potential subject, the research cannot instead be performed with competent persons, and the research entails only minimal risk and minimal burden.

28. When a potential research subject who is deemed incompetent is able to give assent to decisions about participation in research, the physician must seek that assent in addition to the consent of the legally authorized representative. The potential subject's dissent should be respected.

29. Research involving subjects who are physically or mentally incapable of giving consent, for example, unconscious patients, may

Protocol No.: xx/xx/xxx   **Status: Final; Version: 1.0**
This document contains confidential information which is the property of (Name of The Sponsor). It is intended for your internal use only. Do not copy, disclose, or circulate externally without written authorization.
Date: ....

be done only if the physical or mental condition that prevents giving informed consent is a necessary characteristic of the research population. In such circumstances the physician should seek informed consent from the legally authorized representative. If no such representative is available and if the research cannot be delayed, the study may proceed without informed consent provided that the specific reasons for involving subjects with a condition that renders them unable to give informed consent have been stated in the research protocol and the study has been approved by a research ethics committee. Consent to remain in the research should be obtained as soon as possible from the subject or a legally authorized representative.

30. Authors, editors and publishers all have ethical obligations with regard to the publication of the results of research. Authors have a duty to make publicly available the results of their research on human subjects and are accountable for the completeness and accuracy of their reports. They should adhere to accepted guidelines for ethical reporting. Negative and inconclusive as well as positive results should be published or otherwise made publicly available. Sources of funding, institutional affiliations and conflicts of interest should be declared in the publication. Reports of research not in accordance with the principles of this Declaration should not be accepted for publication.

C. ADDITIONAL PRINCIPLES FOR MEDICAL RESEARCH COMBINED WITH MEDICAL CARE

31. The physician may combine medical research with medical care only to the extent that the research is justified by its potential preventive, diagnostic or therapeutic value and if the physician has good reason to believe that participation in the research study will not adversely affect the health of the patients who serve as research subjects

32. The benefits, risks, burdens and effectiveness of a new intervention must be tested against those of the best current proven intervention, except in the following circumstances:

  • The use of placebo, or no treatment, is acceptable in studies where no current proven intervention exists; or
  • Where for compelling and scientifically sound methodological reasons the use of placebo is necessary to determine the efficacy or safety of an intervention and the patients who receive placebo

Protocol No.: xx/xx/xxx   **Status: Final; Version: 1.0**
This document contains confidential information which is the property of (Name of The Sponsor). It is intended for your internal use only. Do not copy, disclose, or circulate externally without written authorization.
Date: ....

or no treatment will not be subject to any risk of serious or irreversible harm. Extreme care must be taken to avoid abuse of this option.

33. At the conclusion of the study, patients entered into the study are entitled to be informed about the outcome of the study and to share any benefits that result from it, for example, access to interventions identified as beneficial in the study or to other appropriate care or benefits.

34. The physician must fully inform the patient which aspects of the care are related to the research. The refusal of a patient to participate in a study or the patient's decision to withdraw from the study must never interfere with the patient-physician relationship.

35. In the treatment of a patient, where proven interventions do not exist or have been ineffective, the physician, after seeking expert advice, with informed consent from the patient or a legally authorized representative, may use an unproven intervention if in the physician's judgment it offers hope of saving life, re-establishing health or alleviating suffering. Where possible, this intervention should be made the object of research, designed to evaluate its safety and efficacy. In all cases, new information should be recorded and, where appropriate, made publicly available.

This document contains confidential information which is the property of (Name of The Sponsor). It is intended for your internal use only. Do not copy, disclose, or circulate externally without written authorization.
Date: ....

Appendix II

INFORMED CONSENT FORM (ICF)

Screening code: [________________________]

Study Title: A randomized, open label, two treatment, two period, two sequence, single dose, crossover, comparative, oral bioavailability study of Montelukast orally disintegrating strip 10 mg (each orally disintegrating strip containing Montelukast Sodium IP equivalent to Montelukast 10 mg) manufactured by the Sponsor with marketed samples of Spiromont 10 mg orally disintegrating strip (each orally disintegrating strip containing Montelukast Sodium IP equivalent to Montelukast 10 mg) manufactured by the company in 16+2 or 24+2 healthy, adult human male subjects under fasting conditions.

Study Number: xx/xx/xxx

Subject's Initials: _______

Subject's Name: ____________________________

Date of Birth/Age/Sex: ___________

Address of the subject: ____

Qualification: ____________________

Annual Income of the subject: _______________________________________

Occupation: Student/ Self-employed/ Service/ Housewife/ Others (please tick the appropriate)

Name and address of the nominee(s) and His relation to the subject (for the purpose of compensation in case of study related injury/death): ____**I hereby willingly agree to participate in the following project: In addition I also declare that I am not an employee or related to any employee of the CRO.**

Please initial by(Subject)

1. I confirm that I have read and understood the information sheet dated ___ for the above study and have had the opportunity to ask questions.   [   ]

2. I understand that my participation in the study is voluntary and that I am free to withdraw at any time, without giving any reason, without my medical care orlegal rights being affected.   [   ]

3. I understand that the Sponsor of the clinical trial, others working on the Sponsor's behalf, the Ethics Committee and the regulatory authorities will not need my permission to look at my health records both in respect of the current study and any further research that may be conducted in relation to it, even if I withdraw from the trial. I agree to this access. However, I understand that my identity will not be revealed in any information released to third parties or published.   [   ]

Protocol No.:xx/xx/xxx; Version: 1.0

4. I agree not to restrict the use of any data or results that arise from this study   [   ]
    provided such a use is only for scientific purpose(s).

5. I agree to take part in the above study.   [   ]

6. I understand that in case of study related injury or death, The Sponsor will   []
    provide complete Medical assistance as well as compensation for the injury or
    death, as per The Government of India, Gazette Notification No. GSR 53 (E)
    dated 30.01.2013 and amended vide GSR 889 (E) dated 12.12.2014.

Signature/Thumb impression of Subject/Legally acceptablerepresentative

Date   **Time :**

Signatory's Name: ____

I confirm that I have read and understood the information regarding the study and that the subject has been explained and has apparently understood this information. The Subject has given his/her consent freely to participate in this study.

Signature of witness

Date:

Name of the Witness:____

Investigator's Declaration:

I declare that the information given in this informed consent document was verbally presented to this subject and that ample time and opportunity were given for this subject/witness to read and understand the contents of this document and enquire about details of the trial and to decide whether or not to participate in the trial. I further certify that I or my authorized designee has discussed the research study with this subject and explained to him or her in non technical terms any risks and adverse reactions that may be expected to occur. I encouraged this subject to ask questions and all questions asked were answered to the satisfaction of the subject. Following this, the subject (and an impartial witness, in case of illiterate subject) signed/attested this informed consent form in my presence.

Protocol No.:xx/xx/xxx; Version: 1.0

____

Signature of the Investigator: **Date:**______________

Study Investigator's Name: ___________________________________

(Copy of the patient information sheet and duly filled Informed Consent Form shall be handed over to the subject or his/ her attendant)

SUBJECT INFORMATION SHEET (SIS)

A RANDOMIZED, OPEN LABEL, TWO TREATMENT, TWO PERIOD, TWO SEQUENCE, SINGLE DOSE, CROSSOVER, COMPARATIVE, ORAL BIOAVAILABILITY STUDY OF MONTELUKAST ORALLY DISINTEGRATING STRIP 10 mg (EACH ORALLY DISINTEGRATING STRIP CONTAINING MONTELUKAST SODIUM IP EQUIVALENT TO MONTELUKAST 10 MG) MANUFACTURED BY THE SPONSOR WITH MARKETED SAMPLES OF SPIROMONT 10 MG ORALLY DISINTEGRATING STRIP (EACH ORALLY DISINTEGRATING STRIP CONTAINING MONTELUKAST SODIUM IP EQUIVALENT TO MONTELUKAST 10 mg) MANUFACTURED BY COMPANY IN 16+2 or 24+2 HEALTHY, ADULT HUMAN MALE SUBJECTS UNDER FASTING CONDITIONS.

Protocol Number: xx/xx/xxx

Protocol Version: 1.0, Dated: ……………..

<u>INFORMATION TO VOLUNTEER</u>

Version 1.0, dated ………………..

Purpose of Research and Benefits

The bioequivalence study in which your participation is proposed, aims to demonstrate the bioequivalence of a single dose of Montelukast orally disintegrating strip 10 mg (each orally disintegrating strip containing Montelukast Sodium IP equivalent to Montelukast 10 mg) manufactured by the Sponsor and a single dose of reference preparation Spiromont 10 mg orally disintegrating strip (each orally disintegrating strip containing Montelukast Sodium IP equivalent to Montelukast 10 mg) manufactured by company under fasting conditions. The knowledge gained from this study would be of benefit to thousands of patients suffering from asthma and also seasonal and perennial allergic rhinitis.

Drug Information

Montelukast: Montelukast is a leukotriene inhibitor. Leukotrienes are chemicals body releases when you breathe in an allergen (such as pollen). These chemicals cause swelling in lungs and tightening of the muscles around airways, which can result in asthma symptoms. Montelukast is used to prevent asthma attacks in adults and children as young as 12 months old. It is also used to relieve runny nose and sneezing caused by allergies in adults and children as young as 6 months old. Montelukast is also used to prevent exercise-induced bronchoconstriction (narrowing of the air passages in the lungs) in adults and teenagers who are at least 15 yrs old and are not already taking this medicine for other conditions. It works by blocking the action of substances in the body that cause the symptoms of asthma and allergic rhinitis.

Rationale of the Montelukast orally disintegrating strip 10 mg

The rationale for using orally disintegrating strip containing montelukast 10 mg is to obtain rapid onset of action with better patient compliance. The patients can take medicine without water. As the drug is directly absorbed into systemic circulation, degradation in gastrointestinal tract and first pass effect can be avoided. Many patients find it difficult to swallow tablets and hard gelatin capsules particularly pediatric and geriatric patients. The knowledge gained from this study would be of benefit to thousands of patients suffering from asthma and also seasonal and perennial allergic rhinitis.

Possible Risks

Common side effects of montelukast areabdominal pain, thirst and headache.

Very rarely there might be dry mouth, diarrhoea, dyspepsia, nausea, vomiting, hepatic disorders, palpitation, oedema, increased bleeding, lack of strength (asthenia), dizziness, hallucinations, abnormal skin sensations (as tingling or tickling or itching or burning), partial loss of sensation (hypoaesthesia), sleep disturbances, abnormal dreams, agitation, aggression, seizures, pain in joints/muscles, itching, and rash.

Study Procedures

Once you are found to be fit in the screening assessments [physical examination, clinical examination (hematology, biochemistry) and serology test], you will be explained about the study title, purpose and background of the study, study procedure, blood sample, restrictions, adverse reactions, risks or discomforts associated with participation in the study, voluntary participation/ refusal, compensation, confidentiality, medical treatment for injury rules and regulations. Safety evaluation will be performed on completion of the study including physical examination and vital signs check. There will be sufficient gap between two periods in order to complete elimination of the drugs from body. Vital signs will be monitored during check-in, before dosing of investigational products and at checkout. You should not take any other medication throughout the study unless you are instructed to do so by the physician at Clinical Pharmacology Unit.

Subjects responsibilities on the participation in the BA/BE Study

You are expected to cooperate fully with the attending doctor. You are also expected to follow the advice given to you by treating doctor and not to deviate from what you have been told to do and what not to do.

Confidentiality

Your medical records will be treated with confidentiality and will be revealed only to other doctors/ scientists/ auditors of this study and if required to the drug regulatory authority. The results of this study may be published in a scientific journal but you will not be identified by name.

Expected duration of participation

The expected duration of participation of the volunteer in this study will be 9 days including a wash out period of 7 days and check in and checkout period of 2 days.

Your participation in the study and your rights

Before agreeing to participate in the present study, it is important that you read and understand the information given in patient information sheet and procedure explained to you. Take time as much you require to take decision to do so. During your participation in the clinical study, you will act as an independent contractor and not as an agent, partner or employee of the CRO. Your participation in this study is voluntary and you may withdraw from the study any time without having to give reasons for the same. In any case, you will be given proper treatment for your condition. Your refusal to participate will not involve any penalty in terms of subsequent participation in research studies. You will agree to cooperate fully with the attending doctor, staff nurse and the phlebotomist. If at any time you feel worse or suffer any other illness, then please inform the coordinator or the staff nurse or the phlebotomist or the attending doctor. If the condition requires any treatment, attending physician will decide and treatment will be provided to you immediately. **If you follow the directions of the physician / in charge of the study and if you are physically injured or dead because of study drug, the sponsor will provide complete medical assistance as well as compensation for the study related injury or death, as per The Government of India, Gazette Notification No. GSR 53 (E) dated 30.01.2013 and amended vide GSR 889 (E) dated 12.12.2014.**

For further questions / problems you may have, you should contact the following person:
(Investigators Name, address & telephone)

Name	Designation	Address	Telephone No.
....	ClinicalInvestigator	....	....
....	Chairman, Ethics Committee	....	....

For any other issues you may have, you should contact the following person:

(Clinical Trial Coordinator's Name, address & telephone)

....

....

Appendix III
SCHEDULE OF STUDY EVENT
Protocol Number: xx/xx/xxx
Drug Name: Montelukast 10 mg
Condition: Fasting

Volunteer screening
(Medical Histories, Demographic data, Physical examination and Laboratory test)

Period I: Subject Check-in at least 11 hr prior to drug administration
(Who meets all the Inclusion Criteria and does not meet any of the Exclusion Criteria)

Volunteer/Subject ID number allotted

Vital signs will be monitored (At each check-in, before dosing and during check-out)

Pre-study Dinner will be served

Indwelling catheter (using heparin-lock technique) will be placed for blood samplingduring pre-dose sample collection. The pre-dose blood sample will be collectedwithin a period of 1 hr prior to the drug administration. The post-dose blood samples will be collected at 0.5, 1.0, 2.0, 2.5, 3.0, 4.0, 6.0, 8.0, 12.0 and 24.0 hrs.

Investigational product will be administered as per randomization schedule at morning in each dosing day in sitting posture (With 240 ± 2 mL water in sitting

Subject well-being questionnaire will be performed (At 1.0 hr, 4.0 hr and 8.0 hr postdose)

Dosing day Lunch, Snacks and Dinner will be served (At 4, 8 and 14 hrpost dose)

Subject Check-out
(24 hr post drug administration)
(Subjects will be informed to come in Period-II Check-in)

Period II: Subject Check-in, Drug Administration, Vital Signs monitoring, Blood sample collection, Meals, Subject well-being questionnaire will be performed as per Period I.

Protocol No.:xx/xx/xxx; Version: 1.0

Appendix-IV

<u>CASE RECORD FORM (CRF)</u>

BIOEQUIVALENCE / BIOAVAILABILITY STUDY

Volunteer'sNo: ....**Study No: xx/xx/xxx**

PRE STUDY DATA

			VITAL SIGNS	
Age (yrs.)			Pulse (BPM)	
Sex	**M/F**		Systolic Blood Pressure (mmHg)	
Height (cms)			Diastolic Blood Pressure (mmHg)	
Weight (Kg)			Temperature (^{o}F)	
BMI (kg/m^2)			Respiratory Rate (per minute)	

Smoking History: Smoker ☐   Non-smoker ☐

If Smoker: Number of Cigarette/Bidi per day:.................

Alcoholic   ☐   Non-alcoholic ☐

If Alcoholic,   Regular ☐ Amount of alcohol intake per day: _____

                 Occasional☐

Medical History :
Surgical History :   H/O allergy:
Family History :
Has the volunteer participated in any drug trial before?   Yes ☐ No ☐
If yes, date on which volunteer last participated in clinical study :
90 day clearance since last clinical study:
Have any problem occurred in previous study :
If yes, specify :

PHYSICAL EXAMINATION

General appearance
Cardiovascular system
Respiratory system
Gastrointestinal system
Central nervous system
Musculoskeletal system
Electrocardiogram (ECG)
Chest X-Ray: Done ☐ Not done ☐ Evaluation:

Signature of the Physician: .... Date: ....

CASE RECORD FORM (CRF)
BIOEQUIVALENCE / BIOAVAILABILITY STUDY
CLINICAL EXAMINATION

Volunteer's No........................ **Study No: xx/xx/xxx**

Sample Collection Date:.................**ReportDate:** ....

Total Count (W. B. C.) -	Normal : 4000-11,000/cu mm.

Differential Count :

Neutrophils : .... (Normal 60 – 70%) Lymphocytes : ....(Normal 25 – 30%)

Monocytes : .... (Normal 00 – 03%)Eosinophil : ....(Normal 00 – 04%)

Basophil : .... (Normal 00 – 0.85%)

Haemoglobin % : (Normal for male : 12.5 – 18 g/mL)	**Blood Glucose :** (Normal Fasting : 76 to 110 mg/dL)
Urea:mg/dL (Normalserum/plasma level – 08 to 45 mg/dL)	**Billirubin :** Direct : mg/dL (Normal 0 to 0.3 mg/dL) Total : mg/dL (Normal 0 to 1.0 mg/dL)
Total Protein :g/dL(Normal 6.2 to 8.5 g/dL)	
Plasma Protein : **Albumin :**g/dL(Normal 3.5 to 5.0 g/dL) **Globulin :**g/dL(Normal 2.8 to 3.8 g/dL) **A/G Ratio :**(Normal 1.0 to 2.0.)	**SGPT :** IU/L(Normal 08 TO 45 IU/L) **Alkaline Phosphate :**IU/L (Normal 30 to 120 IU/L) **Australian Antigen (Hbs Ag):**
VDRL :	**HIV :**
Creatinine: mg/dL (Normal 0.7 to 1.4 mg/dL)	**Cholesterol:**mg/dL (Normal 130 to 240 mg/dL)
Na $^+$: mEq/L (Normal 135 to 150 mEq/L)	**K $^+$:** mEq/L (Normal 3.5 to 5.2 mEq/L)
Urine R/E	
Comment:	

Signature of the Pathologist/ Date: ....

Protocol No.:xx/xx/xxx; Version: 1.0

CASE RECORD FORM (CRF)
VITAL SIGN AND WELL-BEING QUESTIONAIRE RECORDING FORM

Protocol No. xx/xx/xxx	Date:	Period No:
Volunteer Code No.: V	Subject No: S	

Record of Vital Signs

Hour	Scheduled Time	Actual Time	Vital Signs				Performed By
			Temperature (°F)	Blood Press (mmHg)	Pulse Rate (/min)	Respiration Rate (/min)	

Subject Well Being Questionnaire

Hour	Scheduled Time	Actual Time	Subject is feeling		Performed By
			OK	Not OK	

Remarks:____

____

Signature of thePhysician:...............   **Date:** ....

CASE RECORD FORM (CRF)

DRUG ADMINISTRATION, WATER RESTRICTION AND MEAL INTAKE DETAILS FORM

Protocol No. xx/xx/xxx	Date:	Period No:
Volunteer Code No.: V	Subject No: S	

WATER RESTRICTION

Before Drug Administration: _______________________

After Drug Administration: _______________________

DRUG ADMINISTRATION

Time of Drug Administration	Drug Code	Administered with	Mouth Check Performed	Administered by

MEAL INTAKE

Meal	Time of Distribution	Remarks	Administered by
Pre-study dayDinner			
Standard breakfast(Study Day)			
Lunch (Study Day)			
Snacks (Study Day)			
Dinner (Study Day)			

Remarks: ____

Signature of the Physician:.................... **Date:** ....

CASE RECORD FORM (CRF)
BLOOD SAMPLING SCHEDULE

Protocol No. xx/xx/xxx	Date:	Period No:
Volunteer Code No.:	Subject No:	

Sample no.	Interval (hrs)	Actual Timing	Sample Code		Volume of Blood	Remark
			Phase I	Phase II		
					5 ml	
					5 ml	
					5 ml	
					5 ml	
					5 ml	
					5 ml	
					5 ml	
					5 ml	
					5 ml	
					5 ml	
					5 ml	
					5 ml	
					5 ml	
					5 ml	
					5 ml	
					5 ml	
					5 ml	
					5 ml	
					5 ml	

Clinical Pharmacologist/ Doctor

....

Technical Advisor

Blood collectors

1.......................................

2...

3..

4...

CASE RECORD FORM (CRF)
ADVERSE EVENT FORM

Study No: xx/xx/xxx   **Date:**..................

Study Drug administered: ....

Patient Details:

Subject No.: .... **Sex:** ....**Age:** ....

Relevant Medical History:

....

....

ADVERSE EVENT		*ADVERSE EVENT*		*ADVERSE EVENT*	
GIDDINESS		RINGING IN EARS		DARK URINE	
DROWISINESS		VERTIGO		PAIN IN ABDOMEN	
FAINTING		SNEEZING		NAUSEA	
LIGHT HEADEDNESS		NASAL CONGESTION		VOMITTING	
HEADACHE		COLD		ALTERED TASTE	
BLURRING		COUGH		DIARRHEA	
COLORED VISION		DRYNESS OF MOUTH		HYPERACIDITY	
DISCOLORED VISION		SKIN RASH		MUSCLE CRAMPS	
DOUBLE VISION		URTICARIA		TREMORS	
DARK SPOTS		ITCHING		TWITCHING	
LIGHT INTOLERANCE		PALPITATION		WEAKNESS	
WATERING OF EYES		DIFFICULTY BREATHING		JOINT PAIN	
ITCHING IN EYES		CHEST PAIN		NO SLEEP	
DRYNESS OF EYES		FREQUENT URINATION		EXCESSIVE SLEEP	
REDNESS OF EYES		URINARY RETENTION		ANY OTHER	
HEARING IMPAIRMENT		BURNING MICTURATION			

Nature of the Adverse Event

.

Adverse event (describe) ....

....

Date of onset. (dd/mm/yy) ....

Time of onset after the consumption of the drug ....

Severity Grade: Mild ☐   Moderate ☐

Severe ☐   Life threatening ☐

Protocol No.:xx/xx/xxx; Version: 1.0

Concomitant Medication prescribed: ....

....

Relation to study drug

☐   Unrelated (Clearly not related to the study drug)

☐   Unlikely (Doubtfully related to the study drug)

☐   Possible (May be related to the study drug)

☐   Probable (Likely related to the study drug)

☐   Definite (Clearly related to the study drug)

Outcome of Adverse Event:

Fatal ☐   Recovered/Resolved ☐

Recovering/Resolving ☐   Not recovered/Not resolved ☐

Unknown ☐

Follow Up details:

Date: ....   Time: ....

Outcome of Adverse Event (on follow up):

Fatal ☐   Recovered/Resolved ☐

Recovering/Resolving ☐   Not   recovered/Not   resolved   ☐

Unknown ☐

Action Taken:

Continued in the current Study   ☐

Withdrawn from the Study   ☐

Unknown   ☐

Signature of the Physician:.................   **Date:** ....

Protocol No.:xx/xx/xxx; Version: 1.0

Appendix-V

TABLE OF STUDY DIET INCLUDING CALORIE BREAK-UP
Protocol Number: xx/xx/xxx
Drug Name: Montelukast 10 mg
Condition: Fasting

	Menu	Qty.	Total (Cal)*
Dinner (Day: Pre-study)	Rice	200gm (±20gm)	305 (±30)
	Dal	160gm (±15gm)	150 (±15)
	Vegetables	1 bowl/140gm	116
	Potato fry	1 cup (small)	121
	Chicken/Egg/Paneer curry	(4pcs/2pcs/8pcs) =1cup	130
	Total		**822 (Approx)**
Lunch (Day: Study Day)	Rice	200gm (±20gm)	305 (±30)
	Dal	160gm (±15gm)	150 (±15)
	Vegetables (fried/curry)	1 bowl	116
	Fish/Mixed-Veg paneer curry	(2pcs/8pcs) 1 bowl	280
	Chutney	2 spoon	40
	Papad	1 pcs	32
	Curd	113gm	116
	Total		**1039(Approx)**
Snacks (Day: Study Day)	Bread	2 slices	108
	Jam	1 tbs	38
	Milk/ Fruit juice	200mL	122
	Boiled Egg/ Milk Cake	1 No/ 1 chunk	77 -80
	Sweets	1 No (50gm)	76
	Total		**421 (Approx)**
Dinner (Day: Study Day)	Rice Or Chapati (6/7 pcs)	185gm (±18gm)	282/280 (±25)
	Dal	100gm (±10gm)	78 (±12)
	Vegetables	1 bowl (140gm)	198
	Meat /Fish/ Paneer curry	(2pcs/2pcs/8pcs)= 1cup	257-260
	Curd	1 No	32
	Papad	113gm	116
	Total		**963 (Approx)**

*   Fish Curry contains 2 pcs of fish of 175gm; Chicken Curry contains 4 pcs of chicken of 180gm with potato;   Meat Curry contains 2pcs of meat of 180gm with potatoand Egg Curry contains 2 boiled eggs with potato.

** 1 small kilocalorie (kcal) is equal to 1 large food calorie (Cal); 1 kcal=1 Cal
    Ref: http://www.rapidtables.com/convert/energy/1-kcal-to-cal.htm

***Standard Diet Habit in the eastern part of India (West Bengal) (Bengali Volunteers).

Appendix-VI
UNDERTAKING BY THE INVESTIGATOR
(Appendix –VI of Schedule-Y)

1	Full Name, address and title of the Principal Investigator, (or Investigator(s) when there is no Principal Investigator)	:	
2	Name & address of the Medical College, Hospital or other facility where the Clinical Trial will be conducted: Education, training and experience that qualify the Investigator for the Clinical Trial (Attach details including Medical Council Registration No, and / or any other statement(s) of qualification(s))	:	
3	Name & address of all clinical laboratory facilities to be used in study.	:	
4	Name & Address of the Ethics Committee that is responsible for approval & continuing review of study.	:	
5	Names of the other members of the Research Team (Co- or sub-Investigators) who will be assisting the Investigator in the conduct of the investigation(s).	:	
6	Protocol Title and Study number (if any) of the clinical trial to be conducted by the Investigator	:	A randomized, open label, two treatment, two period, two sequence, single dose, crossover, comparative, oral bioavailability study of Montelukast orally disintegrating strip 10 mg (each orally disintegrating strip containing Montelukast Sodium IP equivalent to Montelukast 10 mg) manufactured by the Sponsor with marketed samples of Spiromont 10 mg orally disintegrating strip (each orally disintegrating strip containing Montelukast Sodium IP equivalent to Montelukast 10 mg)manufactured by in 16+2 or 24+2 healthy, adult human male subjects under fasting conditions.
			Study No. xx/xx/xxx

COMMITMENTS

   (i)   I have reviewed the clinical protocol and agree that it contains all the necessary information to conduct the study. I will not begin the study until all necessary ethics committee and regulatory approvals have been obtained.

   (ii)   I agree to conduct the study in accordance with the current protocol. I will not implement any deviation from or changes of the protocol without agreement by the sponsor and prior review and documented approval / favorable opinion from the ethics committee about the amendment, except where necessary to eliminate an immediate hazard to the trial subjects or when the changes involved are logistical or administrative in nature.

   (iii)   I agree to personally conduct and / or supervise the clinical trial at my site.

   (iv)   I agree to inform all subjects that the drugs are being used for investigational purposes and I will ensure that the requirements relating to obtaining informed consent and ethics committee review and approval specified in the GCP guidelines are met.

   (v)   I agree to report to the sponsor all adverse experiences that occurred in the course of investigation in accordance with the regulatory and GCP guidelines.

   (vi)   I have read and understood the information in the investigator's brochure, including the potential risks and side effects of the drug.

   (vii)   I agree to ensure that all associates, colleagues and employees assisting in the conduct of the study are suitably qualified and experienced and they have been informed about their obligations in meeting their commitments in the trial.

   (viii)   I agree to maintain adequate and accurate records and to make those records available for audit / inspection by the sponsor, ethics committee, licensing authority or their authorized representatives, in accordance with regulatory and GCP provisions. I will fully cooperate with any study related audit conducted by regulatory officials or authorized representatives of the sponsor.

   (ix)   I agree to promptly report to the ethics committee all changes in the clinical trial activities and all unanticipated problems involving risks to human subjects or others.

   (x)   I agree to inform all unexpected serious adverse events to the sponsor as well as the ethics committee within 24 hours of their occurrences.

   (xi)   I will maintain confidentiality of the identification of all participating study patients and assure security and confidentiality of study data.

   (xii)   I agree to comply with all other requirements, guidelines, and statutory obligations as applicable to clinical investigators participating in clinical trials.

....

Signature of Investigator   **Date &Stamp**

Appendix-VII

Serious Adverse Event (SAE) Report Form

1. *Basic Information*

Protocol No	xx/xx/xxx
Protocol Title	A randomized, open label, two treatment, two period, two sequence, single dose, crossover, comparative, oral bioavailability study of Montelukast orally disintegrating strip 10 mg (each orally disintegrating strip containing Montelukast Sodium IP equivalent to Montelukast 10 mg) manufactured by the Sponsor with marketed samples of Spiromont 10 mg orally disintegrating strip (each orally disintegrating strip containing Montelukast Sodium IP equivalent to Montelukast 10 mg)manufactured by company in 16+2 or 24+2 healthy, adult human male subjects under fasting conditions.

Generic name of the Drug:	Dosage form:	Frequency:
Indication:	Strength:	Route of administration:
Start date and time of treatment:	End date and time of treatment:	
Concomitant medications:		

IRB		Subject Participated.	
Study start date		Anticipated end date	

2. *Serious Adverse Events*

Date of serious adverse event:	_____ / _____ / _____
Location of SAE:	
Was this an unexpected adverse event?	Yes [ ] No [ ]
Brief description of subject(s)	*Name of the subject:* ___________ *Initials:* _______ *Sex:* M/F *Age:* __________ *Weight:* _________ *Height:* __________ Diagnosis:
Brief description of the nature of the serious adverse event:	
Frequency	*One episode* *Intermittent* *Continuous*

3.Category (Outcome) of the serious adverse event

    [ ] *death*
    [ ] disability/incapacity
    [ ] life-threatening
    [ ] congenital anomaly/birth defect
    [ ] hospitalization-initial or prolonged
    [ ] required intervention to prevent permanent impairment
    [ ] other

Protocol No.:xx/xx/xxx; Version: 1.0

4. *Suspected relationship of serious adverse event:*

      [ ] 1 = unrelated (clearly not related to the research)

      [ ] 2 = unlikely (doubtfully related to the research)

      [ ] 3 = possible (may be related to the research)

      [ ] 4 = probable (likely related to the research)

      [ ] 5 = definite (clearly related to the research)

5. *Other details*

Have similar adverse events occurred on this protocol?	Yes [ ] No [ ] If "Yes", how many? _____ Please Describe:
What steps do you plan to take as a result of the adverse event reported above? Provide documentation to the IRB for review and approval of any of the steps checked below.	[ ] no action required [ ] amend consent document [ ] amend protocol [ ] inform current subjects [ ] terminate or suspend protocol [ ] other, describe:
Information for all subjects/ study design:	
Concomitant medication:	

Report by		
Name and Address	**Signature**	**Date**
Phone: **Occupation:**		

Details of the	Name: _____________________ Phone no._________________
Investigator:	Email._____________________ Fax.: __________________

Investigator's signature:	***Date:***

Appendix-VIII
Utilization Break-Up of Drugs

For 16+2 Volunteers

S. No	Items	Test	Reference
a.	Volunteer Consumption (16+2) for BA/BE Study	18	18
b.	*In-Vitro* Dissolution Study	6	6
c.	Archiving & for 2 yrs Emergency & Repeat Study Uses	20 (at least)	20 (at least)
	Total	44	44

For 24+2 Volunteers

S.No.	Items	Test	Reference
a.	Volunteer Consumption (24+2) for BA/BE Study	26	26
b.	*In-Vitro* Dissolution Study	6	6
c.	Archiving & for 2 yrs Emergency & Repeat Study Uses	20 (at least)	20 (at least)
	Total	50	50

VALIDATION OF A LIQUID CHROMATOGRAPHY MASS SPECTROMETRY METHOD FOR THE DETERMINATION OF MONTELUKAST IN HUMAN PLASMA

Method Validation Protocol
MV Protocol Number: MVP- xx/xx/xxx
Status: Final; Version: 1.0
Date: xxxxx

Study Protocol Number: xx/xx/xx, Version: 1.0
Date: xxxxx

Protocol Prepared by:
………………..

Protocol Approved by:

………………….

Sponsor

…………………………..
………………..

Name of CRO & Address

…………………………………
……………………….

1.0   Authentication
1.1   Bio Analytical Declaration

We, the undersigned, authenticate that we have reviewed this protocol thoroughly and have evaluated the same.

Research Associate
(Name, Signature & Date)

Research Assistant
(Name, Signature & Date)

Approval

I, the undersigned approve that I have thoroughly reviewed this protocol for anomalies and compliance and evaluated the scientific validity of the statements in this protocol and to the best of my knowledge and judgment this protocol is scientifically valid.

Head – Bio-Analytical
(Name, Signature & Date)

Technical Advisor/ Director
(Name, Signature & Date)

1.2   Quality Assurance Declaration

The protocol is verified for compliance with Good Laboratory Practice regulations and implemented Standard Operating Procedures by the Quality Assurance unit of CRO.

Head, Quality Assurance (QA)
(Name, Signature & Date)

2.0 Method Validation Schedule

Schedule	Timelines
Method Validation	
Preparation of Method validation Report	
Review of Method validation Report by Head- BA	
QA Review	

3.0 List of Abbreviations

AR	:	Analytical Reagent
BA	:	Bio-analytical
CAL	:	Calibration Standard
g	:	Gram
GR	:	General Reagent Grade
HPLC	:	High Performance Liquid Chromatography
HQC	:	High Quality Control
IS	:	Internal Standard
LQC	:	Lower Quality Control
LR	:	Laboratory Reagent Grade
M	:	Method
mg	:	Milligram
mL	:	Milliliter
MQC	:	Middle Quality Control
ng	:	Nanogram
No.	:	Number
P&A	:	Precision and Accuracy
QA	:	Quality Assurance
QC	:	Quality Control
RA	:	Research Associate
SOP	:	Standard Operating Procedure
TBME	:	Tert-Butyl Methyl Ether

4.0   Description of Materials

Test Article: Refer Annexure I for the certificate of analysis

Working Standard	Montelukast
Batch No	------
Expiry	------
Purity	------
Storage	------
Mol. Wt.	------
Source	------

Internal Standard: Refer Annexure II for the certificate of analysis

Working Standard	------
Batch No	------
Expiry	------
Purity	------
Storage	------
Mol. Wt.	------
Source	------

5.0   Objective

To describe the process as well as validate a bio analytical method for estimation of montelukast in human plasma using as an internal standard (IS).

6.0 Scope

This procedure is applicable for the analysis of montelukast in human plasma.

7.0 Study Personnel Name and Roles

S. No	Personnel Name	Roles
1.		Review of Final Protocols
2.		Bulk Spiking, Sample Processing, Instrument Operation
3.		Sample Processing

8.0   Procedure

8.1   Experimental

8.1.1 Chemical, Reagents and Matrix

Chemical	Reagents	Matrix
Montelukast (Working Standard)		
Internal Standard		Blank Human Plasma
Formic Acid (AR Grade)		
Water – HPLC Grade		

8.1.2 Equipment

Equipment	Make	Serial Number
HPLC pump	Shimadzu LC20AD	L20104717593
HPLC Autosampler	Shimadzu SIL20AC	L20354701578
Triple Quadrupole Mass Spectrometer API 2000	AB Sciex Instruments	B018520603
Deep Freezer (-20°C)	Celfrost	091131273
Centrifuge	REMI group	CPLC-1503
Evaporator	Home made	-
pH meter	Sartorius	PB-11
Top loading balance	Sartorius	17505932

8.2   Preparation of Solutions

8.2.1 Preparation of Mobile Phase A: Water containing 0.1% Formic Acid

8.2.2 Preparation of Mobile Phase B: Methanol containing 0.1% Formic Acid

8.3   Preparation of Stock Solution
8.3.1 Montelukast Stock Solution (W/V)
8.3.2 ISTD Stock Solution (W/V)

8.4   Preparation of CC Standard and QC Standard Samples

8.4.1 Preparation of Calibration Curve (CC)

8.4.1.1   Preparation of Blank Sample: Matrix is processed without IS & analyzed.

8.4.1.2   Preparation of Zero Sample: Matrix is processed with IS & analyzed.

8.4.1.3   Preparation of Standard Stock Solution (w/v): Prepare as per 8.3.1.

8.4.1.4   Preparation of Intermediate Concentration: Add 2 ml of Montelukast 1 mg/mL stock solution 8ml methanol to get the concentration of 200 µg/mL

Table A Preparation of Intermediate Concentration

Stock Conc. (µg /mL)	Stock Aliquot (mL)	Diluent Added (mL)	Final Volume (mL)	Final Conc. (µg/mL)
…..	…..	…..	…..	…..
…..	…..	…..	…..	…..

8.4.1.5 Preparation of Stock Dilutions: Prepare stock dilutions of Montelukast in the concentration of 160 µg/mL to 1.25 µg/mL using intermediate starting concentration 200 µg/mL and further serial dilution.

Table B. Preparation of Montelukast Stock Dilutions

Stock Conc. (µg/mL)	Stock volume Taken (µL)	Solvent added (µL)	Final Conc. (µg/mL)
…..	…..	…..	…..
…..	…..	…..	…..

Complete the "Stock Dilution Form"

8.4.1.4 Drug spiking in blank Human plasma for Calibration Curve: Transfer 100µl of each of the corresponding concentrations of the above described stock dilutions of montelukast into 900µl blank Human plasma to achieve calibration concentration points given below.

Table-C Preparation of Montelukast Calibration Solution in Spiked Plasma

Stock Concentrations of Montelukast (µg/mL)	Montelukast Concentration in spiked plasma (µg/mL)	Spiked Plasma Concentration ID
…..	…..	…..
…..	…..	…..

Concentrations in plasma represent uncorrected concentrations. True concentrations may vary as per potency and the actual amount weighed. Pipette 0.180 mL blank human plasma aliquot of each calibration spiked standard into polypropylene-capped tubes and freeze at -20°C until analysis.

8.4.2 Quality Control (QC) Samples

8.4.2.1 Preparation of Stock Dilutions

Prepare QC stock dilutions of montelukast in a concentration using diluents as described in the Table D below.

Table D Preparation of Quality Control Stock Dilution

Stock Montelukast Conc (µg/mL)	Stock Aliquot	Diluent Added (mL)	Final Volume (mL)	Final Conc.
…..	…..	…..	…..	…..
…..	…..	…..	…..	…..

Complete the "Stock Dilution Form"

8.4.2.2 Spiking of Plasma for Quality Control Samples: Transfer 100 µl of each of the corresponding concentrations of the above described stock dilutions into 900 µl blank Human plasma to achieve HQC, MQC and LQC respectively.

Table E Preparation of Montelukast QC Concentration in Spiked Plasma

Stock Conc. (µg/mL)	Final C onc. in spiked plasma (µg/mL)	Spiked Plasma Conc. ID
…..	…..	…..
…..	…..	…..
…..	…..	…..

Concentrations in plasma represent uncorrected concentrations. True concentrations may vary as per potency and the actual amount weighed. Pipette 180 µL aliquot of each quality control samples into polypropylene-capped tubes and freeze at -20°C until analysis.

8.5   Bio Analytical Method

8.5.1 Sample Preparation

Withdraw the spiked blank human plasma samples from the deep freezer and allow them to thaw at room temperature

Add 300 µL of aliquot and 30 µL internal standard (…… 2 µg/mL) into 15 mL centrifuge tubes and vortex for 30 seconds

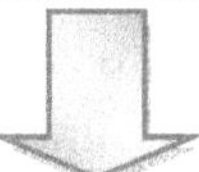

Add upto 1.5 mL of TBME and vortex for 10 minutes

Centrifuge at 5000 rpm for 10 minutes

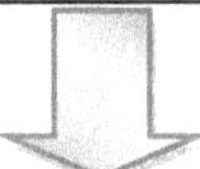

Separate 1 mL of supernatant organic layer and evaporate at 45°C for 10 minutes under N_2 atmosphere

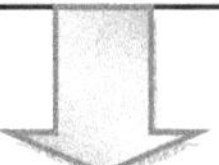

Reconstitute with 200 µL of 1:1 MeOH: H_2O and inject sample into LC-MS/MS

8.5.2 Chromatographic Conditions

Column	------	
Mobile Phase	A:	and B:
Flow rate	------	
Injection volume	------	
Total run time(min)	------	
Auto sampler Temperature	------	
Retention Time (min)	Montelukast:	and Internal Std :

The mobile phase and the flow rate may be modified to optimize the chromatographic response. The retention times listed should not be considered as method specifications but as assay method parameters.

8.5.3 Multiple Reaction Monitoring (MRM) Conditions

Compound	Q1	Q3	Dwell Time	DP	CE	CXP
Montelukast	.....	.....	.....	.....	.....	.....
Internal Std	.....	.....	.....	.....	.....	.....
DP = Declustering Potential; CE = Collision Energy; CXP = Collision Cell Exit Potential						

9.0   Validation Parameters

9.1   Selectivity

A minimum of six matrix lots will be used and screened for selectivity out of which one is hemolytic and one is lipemic. From each lot of matrix, a blank and LLOQ sample is spiked and processed as per the method procedure. The processed samples were injected and analyzed. The interference in the blank matrix will be evaluated by comparing the response at the retention time of analytic and internal standard against the response of analyte and internal standard in the extracted LLOQ samples.

Acceptance Criteria:
- Response of the interfering peak at the retention time of analyte should be ≤20% of mean response of analyte(s) in LLOQ concentration.
- For internal standard, the response of the interfering peak at the R.T of IS should be ≤5% of mean response of IS in LLOQ sample.

9.2   Back Calculated Concentrations for Calibration Curve Standards:

Back calculations will be made from the calibration curves to determine concentrations of calibration standards (Table B) of the analyte.

Any one of LLOQ and ULOQ (submitted in duplicate) should compulsorily pass and no two consequent points should fail. All the calibration curve points, HQC, MQC and LQC samples should be within ±15% of the specified concentrations, except for the LLOQ within ± 20%. 75% of the calibration standards should be within the acceptance range including the lowest and highest calibration standard. While considering the individual QC level a minimum of 50% should be within acceptance range. Overall a minimum of 67% of the QC's in the P&A batch should be within acceptance range. Remaining 33% of the QC samples (not all the replicates at the same concentration) may be above 15% provided the mean accuracy values are within the acceptance range.% CV should be within ±15% at HQC, MQC, LQC and ±20% LLOQ QC levels.

9.3   Precision and Accuracy

9.3.1 Within–Batch Accuracy and Precision

The within–batch accuracy and precision shall be assessed by the repeated analysis of blood samples containing different concentrations on three P & A batches using 2 analysts on separate occasions. A single run consists of a calibration curve plus 6 replicates of the LQC, MQC and HQC samples in singlets. In Calibration curve LLOQ and ULOQ samples alone are run in duplicates.

9.3.2 Between-Batch Accuracy and Precision

The between–batch accuracy and precision shall be assessed by the repeated analysis of precision and accuracy batches containing different concentrations of drug on two consecutive days. Two precision and accuracy batches shall be carried out on a single day and the third batch on the other day. A single run consists of a calibration curve plus 6 replicates of the LQC, MQC and HQC in singlets. In Calibration curve LLOQ and ULOQ samples alone are run in duplicates.

9.3.3 Run Acceptance Criteria

Any one of LLOQ and ULOQ should compulsorily pass and no two consequent points should fail. All the calibration curve points, HQC, MQC and LQC samples should be within ±15% of the specified concentrations, except for the LLOQ within ± 0%. While considering the individual QC level a minimum of 50% should be within acceptance range. Overall a minimum of 67% of the QC's in the P&A batch should be within acceptance range. Remaining 33% of the QC samples (not all the replicates at the same concentration) may be above 15% provided the mean accuracy values are within the acceptance range. % CV is within ±15% at HQC, MQC, LQC and ±20% LLOQ QC levels.

9.4   Recovery

Six replicates of extracted HQC, MQC and LQC are prepared as per the method procedure. Freshly prepared aqueous QC samples based on recovery along with the extracted QC samples are injected. The mean peak area response of the extracted samples is compared with the mean peak area response of the aqueous samples. The mean of % recovery, standard deviation and %CV are calculated for each level and the global mean % recovery of analyte and internal standards are calculated. % Recovery for analyte(s) and IS(s) should not be more than 115% and % CV of area at different concentrations (i.e., HQC, MQC and LQC) should be <15%. % CV of Global Recovery should be ±20%.

9.5 Stock Solution Stability

9.5.1 Short-term Stock Solution Stability

Short term stock solution stability for the analyte and the internal standard shall be assessed after 6 hours at room temperature along with freshly prepared stock solution at middle level quality control concentration. The mean peak response of the "0" hour and "n" hour stock solution(s) should be within the range of 90-110%.

9.5.2 Long-term Stock Solution Stability: Long term stock solution stability for the analyte and the internal standard shall be assessed for a minimum of 3 days or for the prescribed time at 2 to 8°C along with freshly prepared stock solution at middle level quality control concentration. The mean peak response of the "0" hour and "n" hour stock solution(s) should be within the range of 90- 110%.

9.6 Freeze Thaw Stability

A calibration curve shall be processed along with 6 replicates of stability samples at low and high QC levels which shall be subjected to four freeze thaw cycles. In first cycle sample shall be frozen at -80°C for 24hours, then it shall be thawed to room temperature until it gets completely thawed. The second cycle and the subsequent cycles shall be further frozen at -80°C for minimum 12 hours and thawed to room temperature. After the 4th cycle the samples shall be analyzed in a single run. The mean concentration obtained for stability QC samples should be 85-115% of nominal concentration of freshly prepared QC samples. The % CV should be within ±15%.

9.7 Matrix Effect

Six different lots of blood shall be processed in duplicates (without spiking analyte and internal standard) as per the extraction procedure and before reconstitution step, the aqueous HQC and LQC samples are spiked with internal standard and analyzed. Aqueous samples shall be prepared based on recovery for both analyte and internal standard at HQC and LQC levels and injected along with the post spiked samples and analyzed to determine the effect of matrix with the analyte or the internal standard. Matrix effect should be within ±15% and 75% of lots used should pass the matrix effect.

10.0 Data Processing

Acquire chromatograms using the computer-based software supplied by AB Sciex Instruments Analyst 1.4.2 by peak area ratio. Determine the standard curve fitting the concentration and response relationship using linear $1/x^2$ weighing and statistical tests for goodness of fit.

$$y = mx+c$$

Where

x = concentration of Montelukast

y = peak area ratio of Montelukast

c = y axis intercept of the calibration curve

11.0 Method Validation Protocol Structure

The method validation shall be performed as per Guidelines for Bioavailability & Bioequivalence Studies published by CDSCO in March 2005.

12.0 Quality Control Role

QC staff will check the Method validation raw data, results, log book entries and related documentation as follows:
- Raw data
- Logbooks and the data
- Weighing, printout
- Documentation of any SOP / protocol deviation.
- Analytical run sequence
- Results table and chromatograms

13.0 Quality Assurance Role

QA staff shall monitor/ inspect and audit the following activities:
- Stock solution preparation.
- Bulk spiking of CCs and QCs
- Forms issue and control
- Inspection during the method validation experiments
- Checking and auditing of raw data entries and assuring that the results are transcribed correctly in the method validation protocol
- QA authentication of Method validation protocol

14.0 Record Keeping

The method validation raw data and chromatograms are compiled and after the approval of QA the files (hard and soft copy) are maintained in the archive for a period of 5 years from the date of signing of the protocol.

15.0 Method Validation Protocol Deviations

Concentrations reflected in the protocol are suggested ranges for Calibration Curve and Quality control samples may be altered to specific needs of the study design. The concentrations should be within the range given in the method validation protocol. The chromatographic parameters and instrumentation parameters may also be optimized to get the specific response for the analytes and internal standard. Apart from this any other deviations from the method validation protocol will be documented in memo to file.

16.0 Health and Safety Requirements

All the personnel involving in sample processing are vaccinated with Hepatitis B vaccine. While processing samples proper personnel protective equipment like, face mask, head caps, gloves, apron are worn to reduce the risk of potentially infectious materials. Fire extinguisher, emergency shower, eye wash fountains are in the lab and periodic functional checks are documented.

17.0 Annexure-I: COA of Montelukast

18.0 Annexure-II: Definitions

Accuracy: Accuracy is the closeness of determined value to the true value. Generally, recovery of added analyte over an appropriate range of concentrations is taken as an indication of accuracy. (The concentration range chosen should bracket the concentration of interest).

Analyte: A specific chemical moiety being measured, which can be intact drug, biomolecule or its derivative, metabolite, and/or degradation product in a biologic matrix.

Analytical run (or batch): A complete set of analytical and study samples with appropriate number of standards and QCs for their validation. Several runs (or batches) may be completed in one day, or one run (or batch) may take several days to complete.

Biological matrix: A discrete material of biological origin that can be sampled and processed in a reproducible manner. Examples are blood, serum, plasma, urine, feces, saliva, sputum, and various discrete tissues.

Blank: A sample of a biological matrix to which no analytes have been added that is used to assess the specificity of the bioanalytical method.

Calibration standard: A biological matrix to which a known amount of analyte has been added or spiked. Calibration standards are used to construct calibration curves from which the concentrations of analytes in QCs and in unknown study samples are determined.

Internal standard: Test compound(s) (e.g. structurally similar analog, stable labeled compound) added to both calibration standards and samples at known and constant concentration to facilitate quantification of the target analyte(s).

Lower limit of quantification (LLOQ): The lowest amount of an analyte in a sample that can be quantitatively determined with suitable precision and accuracy.

Matrix effect: The direct or indirect alteration or interference in response due to the presence of unintended analytes (for analysis) or other interfering substances in the sample.

Method: A comprehensive description of all procedures used in sample analysis.

Precision: The closeness of agreement (degree of scatter) between a series of measurements obtained from multiple sampling of the same homogenous sample under the prescribed conditions.

Processed: The final extract (prior to instrumental analysis) of a sample that has been subjected to various manipulations (e.g., extraction, dilution, concentration).

Recovery: The extraction efficiency of an analytical process, reported as a percentage of the known amount of an analyte carried through the sample extraction and processing steps of the method.

Reproducibility: The precision between two laboratories. It also represents precision of the method under the same operating conditions over a short period of time.

Sample: A generic term encompassing controls, blanks, unknowns & processed samples, as described below:

Blank: A sample of a biological matrix to which no analytes have been added that is used to assess the specificity of the bioanalytical method.

Quality control sample (QC): A spiked sample used to monitor the performance of a bioanalytical method and to assess the integrity and validity of the results of the unknown samples analyzed in an individual batch.

Unknown: A biological sample that is the subject of the analysis.

Selectivity: The ability of the bioanalytical method to measure and differentiate the analytes in the presence of components that may be expected to be present. These could include metabolites, impurities, degradants, or matrix components.

Stability: The chemical stability of an analyte in a given matrix under specific conditions for given time intervals.

Standard curve: The relationship between the experimental response value and the analytical concentration (also called a calibration curve).

System suitability: Determination of instrument performance (e.g., sensitivity and chromatographic retention) by analysis of a reference standard prior to running the analytical batch.

Upper limit of quantification (ULOQ): The highest amount of an analyte in a sample that can be quantitatively determined with precision and accuracy.

Validation: Establishment of all validation parameters to apply to sample analysis for the bioanalytical method for each analyte.

19.0 Annexure-III: List of Formulae Used

Accuracy:

$$\% \text{ Nominal} = \frac{\text{Mean Concentration}}{\text{Actual Concentration}} \times 100$$

Precision:

$$\%CV = \frac{\text{Standard Deviation}}{\text{Mean}} \times 100$$

Recovery:

$$\% \text{ Recovery} = \frac{\text{Mean Area of Extracted}}{\text{Mean Area of Un-extracted}} \times 100$$

$$\text{Total Mean Recovery \%} = \frac{\% \text{ Recovery of (LQC+MQC+HQC)}}{3} \times 100$$

Stability:

$$\% \text{ Stability} = \frac{\text{Average Area of n Hrs}}{\text{Average Area of 0 Hr}} \times 100$$

Matrix Effect:

$$\% \text{ of Matrix Effect} = \frac{\text{Extracted Area value}}{\text{Mean Area of Un-extracted}} \times 100$$

Chapter 6

Contents of a BE Study Report

MAIN STUDY REPORT

I. Brief Description of the Study

***Study Title** (Protocol No. xx/xx/xxx, Version No. 1.0, Date: xxxxx)*
A randomized two way, two periods, two treatments cross over bioequivalence study of test preparation, Montelukast Orally Disintegrating Strip (ODS) 10 mg (each orally disintegrating strip containing Montelukast Sodium IP equivalent to Montelukast 10 mg), manufactured by Sponsor, in comparison with Spiromont 10 mg Orally Disintegrating Strip (ODS) (each orally disintegrating strip containing Montelukast Sodium IP equivalent to Montelukast 10 mg), manufactured by Sponsor, in 16+2 healthy male, adult, human volunteers under fasting condition.

Details of Person-in-Charge and Address

- Institution
- Principal/ Medical/Clinical Investigator
- Clinical Laboratory
- Analytical Laboratory
- Data Management, Pharmacokinetics and Statistical Analysis
- Other Investigator(s) and Study Personnel

Start and End Date of Clinical and Analytical Study

Clinical Study	
Period I:	**Period II:**
Start Date: 25/07/2017	Start Date: 02/08/2017
Stop Date: 26/07/2017	Stop Date: 03/08/2017
Analytical Study	
Method Validation	**Volunteer Plasma**
Start Date: 21/07/2017	Start Date: 07/08/2017
End Date : 06/08/2017	End Date: 10/08/2017

Signature of Investigator(s), (Medical Writer, QA Manager – if applicable) and Date

II. Summary of the Study

On the basis of the pharmacokinetic parameters C_{max}, t_{max}, AUC_{o-t}, and AUC_{0-inf}, $t_{1/2}$ and k_{el} studied, it can be concluded that the test preparation, Montelukast (ODS) 10mg mfg. by The Sponsor is bioequivalent with the reference preparation, Spiromont 10 mg (ODS), manufactured by the sponsor. The relative bioavailability of the test preparation, Montelukast (ODS) 10 mg, was 101.06% with that of the reference preparation, Spiromont 10 mg (ODS).

III. Table of Contents

Sl.	Particulars
I.	Brief Description of the Study
II	Summary of the Study
III.	Table of Contents
1.	Aims & Objectives
2.	Subjects
3.	Materials & Methods
3.1	Study Design
3.2	Product Information
3.3	Dose
3.4	Blood Collection
4.	LC-MS/MS Analysis
5.	Pharmacokinetic Variables Studied
6.	Results
6.1	Pharmacokinetic Parameters
6.2	Adverse Reaction
7.	Discussion
8.	Conclusion

Table No.	Particulars
1.	Demographic Data
2.	Randomization
3.	Plasma Concentration Table of Reference Preparation (A1)
4.	Plasma Concentration Table of Test Preparation (A2)
5.	Pharmacokinetic Parameters of Reference & Test Preparations in 24 Volunteers
6.	Summary of Pharmacokinetic parameters of Reference & Test Preparations

Sr. No.	Particulars
I	(a)Plasma Concentration Vs Time Graphs of 16 Volunteers (b)Mean Plasma Concentration Vs Time Graph
II	SAS output of Statistical Parameters, 90% confidence interval & Anova
III	Protocol & Approval
IV	Method Validation Report
V	(a)Volunteers ICFs (Informed Consent Forms) (b)Volunteers Check-in, Check –out, Cloth Register
VI	Selection and Timing of Dose for each subject (CRF 4)
VII	Individual Laboratory Measurements (CRF 2)
VIII	Vital Signs (CRF 1)
IX	Data Quality Assurance
X	Signature of principal or coordinating investigator
XII	List of IECs or IRBs (plus the name of the committee Chair if required by regulatory authority) - Representative written information for patient and sample consent forms
XIII	Comparison of Dissolution Profiles
XIV	COA (Certificate of Analysis)
XV	Chromatograms of Method Validation & Volunteer Plasma Samples

1. Aims and Objectives

The aim and the objective of the present study was to evaluate the pharmacokinetic parameters and to compare the bioequivalence of Montelukast (ODS) 10 mg (each orally disintegrating strip containing Montelukast Sodium IP equivalent to Montelukast 10 mg) with Spiromont 10 mg (ODS) (each orally disintegrating strip containing Montelukast Sodium IP equivalent to Montelukast 10 mg) in 16+2 healthy human volunteers in a randomized, two way complete crossover design.

2. Subjects

Subjects were adult, human, healthy male volunteers the mean age 32.72 ± 4.85 yrs and mean weight 55.89 ± 7.39 kg (Table 1), selected from the panel of volunteers. Volunteers were screened for inclusion in the study within 21 days before the commencement of the study. They fulfilled the selection criteria as per the protocol submitted earlier (Annexure-I). Before admission to the study each subject was informed of the nature and the risks of the study and a written informed consent was obtained from the volunteers. They were allocated to the treatment A1 / A2 (Reference or Test preparation) in accordance with the randomization code (Table 2).

3. Materials and Methods

3.1 Study Design: This was a single dose, randomized, two treatment and two-way cross over study, with at least a washout period of 7 days between the two dosing sessions. In each dosing session, volunteers received either of the Test or the Reference preparation of Montelukast only on the study day at a fixed time.

3.2 Product Information

Reference Preparation (A1)

Spiromont 10 mg Orally Disintegrating Strip

Mfg by: XXXXXXX

Batch No.: FP97D601

Mfg Date: 04/2016

Exp. Date: 03/2018

Test Preparation (A2)

Montelukast Orally Disintegrating Strip 10 mg

Mfg. by: Sponsor

Batch No.: SCB-MS-010-FRD04

Mfg. Date: 04/17

3.3 Dose: With both the preparation, the dose was one orally disintegrating strip containing Montelukast Sodium IP equivalent to Montelukast 10 mg.

3.4 Blood Collection: All the volunteers assembled in CPU at 5.00 am on the study day of each session, after overnight fasting of 10 hrs. Their TPR, BP was recorded and an indwelling intravenous catheter was introduced with strict aseptic precautions in the suitable vein for blood collection. They received either of the study preparations according to their randomization schedule at 6.00 am.

A total of 11 blood samples of each volunteer were collected at 0 hr. (before drug administration) and 0.5, 1.0, 2.0, 2.5 , 3.0, 4.0, 6.0, 8.0 , 12.0 , 24.0 hrs.(after drug administration) in the test tubes with EDTA at each time point. Lunch, snacks and dinner were provided after 4 hrs, 8 hrs, and 14 hrs respectively after drug ingestion. On the study days volunteers were permitted normal activities, excluding strenuous exercise.

Collected blood samples were centrifuged immediately & plasma was separated and stored frozen at –20°C with appropriate labeling of volunteer code no with study date and collection time. Abnormal signs / symptoms were monitored, during the study period and for one week after the study period and if noticed, their details were entered in the case report sheets and tabulated at the end of the study.

4. LCMS/MS Analysis

Samples were analyzed by LC-MS/MS after extracting the drug from plasma and injecting it on the LC-MS/MS column for chromatographic analysis. The blood plasma concentration of the volunteers for Reference and Test preparation are tabulated in Table 3 & Table 4.

5. Pharmacokinetic Variables Studied

Plasma levels of Montelukast for every volunteer at each time point were plotted to obtain Time-Plasma concentration curves for the study preparations. The mean parameters of Bioavailability for this single dose study were: -

C_{max} (Maximum Plasma Concentration)

t_{max} (Time to Maximum Plasma Concentration)

$AUC_{(0-24)}$ (The area under plasma concentration time curve)

$AUC_{(0-inf)}$ (The area under plasma concentration time curve 0 to infinity)

$t_{1/2}$ (Elimination half-life)

K_{el} (Elimination rate constant)

6. Results

6.1 Pharmacokinetic Parameters: Administration of the Reference preparation, Spiromont 10 mg (ODS) (each orally disintegrating strip containing Montelukast Sodium IP equivalent to Montelukast 10 mg), as a single dose in the fasting state produced the maximum plasma concentration of 443.86 ± 117.44 ng/ml (C_{max}) at the time 3.03 ± 0.76 hr (t_{max}) whereas administration of the Test preparation, Montelukast (ODS)   10 mg (each orally disintegrating strip containing Montelukast sodium IP equivalent to montelukast 10 mg), as a single dose in the fasting state produced the maximum plasma concentration 450.14 ± 74.24 ng /ml (C_{max}) at the time 3.22 ± 1.00 hr (t_{max}) (Table 5 & 6).

Administration of the Reference preparation, Spiromont 10 mg (ODS), produced the area under plasma concentration time curve (AUC_{0-24}) 2627.21 ± 1046.19 ng.hr./ml, whereas administration of the Test preparation, Montelukast (ODS) 10 mg, produced the area under plasma concentration curve (AUC_{0-24}) 2655.18 ± 744.94 ng.hr./ml (Table 5 & 6).

When administered as a single dose, in the fasting state, the Reference preparation, Spiromont 10 mg (ODS), produced the area under plasma concentration time curve up to infinity ($AUC_{0-\alpha}$) 2690.44 ± 1059.61 ng.hr./ml, whereas administration of the Test preparation, Montelukast (ODS) 10 mg, produced area under plasma concentration time curve up to infinity ($AUC_{0-\alpha}$) 2745.26 ± 780.95 ng.hr./ml (Table 5 & 6).

Administration of the Reference preparation, Spiromont 10 mg (ODS), produced the plasma elimination half-life, ($t_{1/2}$) 3.937 ± 0.476 hr whereas administration of the Test preparation, Montelukast (ODS) 10 mg, produced the plasma elimination half-life ($t_{1/2}$) 4.102 ± 0.900 hr (Table 5 & 6). Administration of the Reference preparation, Spiromont 10 mg (ODS), produced the plasma elimination constant (K_{el}) 0.179 ± 0.028 hr^{-1}, whereas administration of the Test preparation, Montelukast (ODS) 10 mg, produced the plasma elimination constant ($K_{el)}$ 0.177 ± 0.041 hr^{-1} (Table 5 & 6).

On the basis of comparison of the AUC_{0-24} of Montelukast, after single dose administration, the relative bioavailability of the Test preparation, Montelukast (ODS) 10 mg was 101.06% with that of the Reference preparation, Spiromont 10 mg (ODS).

6.2 Adverse Reactions: None of the volunteers complained of any adverse reaction on the pharmacokinetic profile days.

7. Discussion

The single dose bioequivalence study of montelukast (ODS) 10 mg was conducted in 16+2 adult healthy, human, male volunteers with two preparations of montelukast. Values of C_{max}, t_{max} and AUC_{0-24}, were comparable for the reference and the test preparation in the fasting state.

Montelukast was detected in plasma from 0.5 hr to about 24.0 hrs for both the preparations. Peak plasma levels of montelukast were achieved 2.0 to 4.0 hrs for both the preparations. The mean peak plasma levels of montelukast with Reference preparation, Spiromont 10 mg (ODS), on the study day ranged between 311.20–621.08 ng/ml. While the test preparation, montelukast (ODS) 10 mg, ranged between 347.87–633.25 ng/ml. On the basis of comparison of the AUC_{0-24} for montelukast after single dose administration, the relative bioavailability of the test preparation, montelukast (ODS) 10 mg was 101.06% with that of the reference preparation, Spiromont 10 mg (ODS).

8. Conclusion

On the basis of the pharmacokinetic parameters studied, it can be concluded that the Test preparation, Montelukast (ODS) 10 mg mfg by the Sponsor is bioequivalent with the Reference preparation, Spiromont 10 mg (ODS).

Technical Advisor /Director   **Clinical Investigator**
(Signature and date)

Results, Tables and Graphs

Table 1 Demographic Data of 16+2 Volunteers

Vol. No.	Sex	Age	Height (cm)	Weight (kg)	BMI (kg/m^2)
1	M	32	171	70	23.94
2	M	37	171	70	23.94
3	M	30	167	51	18.29
4	M	30	168	55	19.49
5	M	27	164	52	19.33
6	M	38	156	55	22.60
7	M	38	176	70	22.60
8	M	28	163	62	23.34
9	M	38	165	51	18.73
10	M	36	161	55	21.22
11	M	30	160	50	19.53
12	M	38	155	52	21.64
13	M	25	162	52	19.81
14	M	35	167	52	18.65
15	M	38	163	51	19.20
16	M	26	154	55	23.19
Mean		**32.72**	**163.83**	**55.89**	**21.01**
S.D.		**4.85**	**6.07**	**7.39**	**2.44**

Table 2 Mode of Treatment

Subject No.	Period I	Period II
1	A2	A1
2	A2	A1
3	A1	A2
4	A1	A2
5	A2	A1
6	A1	A2
7	A1	A2
8	A1	A2
9	A1	A2
10	A2	A1
11	A2	A1
12	A1	A2
13	A2	A1
14	A1	A2
15	A1	A2
16	A2	A1
A1 – Reference Preparation; A2 – Test Preparation		

No.	0	0.5	1.0	2.0	2.5	3.0	4.0	6.0	8.0	12.0	24.0
1	0	89.18	97.79	205.36	**478.59**	339.84	283.69	218.12	158.06	25.47	14.42
2	0	76.30	146.35	251.80	265.41	**406.59**	214.77	157.28	45.81	31.91	8.70
3	0	130.20	199.22	**311.20**	266.50	179.69	105.81	77.61	55.75	38.61	8.67
4	0	129.99	255.46	322.97	351.30	430.87	**496.29**	361.45	102.87	42.60	17.63
5	0	26.21	51.02	282.34	382.17	**471.55**	397.33	365.09	302.85	49.26	1.88
6	0	127.25	259.49	306.16	336.49	407.64	**495.45**	369.43	104.94	39.46	15.40
7	0	47.55	86.35	172.28	**362.28**	291.67	256.98	198.84	127.50	17.76	12.22
8	0	59.30	112.65	191.52	219.73	**360.90**	186.89	132.62	43.01	29.39	7.15
9	0	30.75	64.16	131.94	**320.62**	258.43	205.08	168.88	120.36	14.77	12.11
10	0	44.32	95.07	189.00	206.58	**316.39**	143.82	113.37	22.63	20.97	5.39
11	0	95.74	225.61	**615.29**	534.02	428.63	314.24	185.74	106.18	48.93	7.19
12	0	77.68	198.99	245.75	327.50	487.63	**621.08**	409.95	292.20	140.34	18.73
13	0	14.02	30.82	175.13	246.59	**324.45**	265.64	237.94	216.67	107.43	12.54
14	0	72.95	135.11	166.80	223.63	288.97	**327.29**	243.13	68.94	26.94	9.04
15	0	85.75	232.88	**591.02**	456.11	383.78	238.43	142.94	90.62	45.03	6.79
16	0	95.36	216.10	382.99	449.89	516.47	**602.77**	419.66	219.48	131.02	15.23
Mean	0	**75.16**	**150.44**	**283.85**	339.21	**368.34**	**322.22**	237.63	**129.87**	**50.62**	**10.82**
S. D.	0	**36.49**	76.45	142.37	100.28	90.54	157.54	112.13	86.22	39.45	4.72
C.V.%	0	**48.55**	50.82	50.16	29.56	24.58	48.89	47.19	66.39	77.94	43.59

Vol. No.	Time (in hours)										
	0	0.5	1.0	2.0	2.5	3.0	4.0	6.0	8.0	12.0	24.0
1	0	50.45	91.94	189.46	**462.04**	366.09	256.49	246.71	126.31	54.35	21.87
2	0	108.78	205.09	250.15	351.85	**517.32**	248.5	200.08	99.77	39.64	10.58
3	0	143.41	232.49	**375.51**	284.63	236.18	145.66	96.11	58.82	43.91	10.94
4	0	150.41	308	351.38	395.28	442.12	**633.25**	429.83	158.93	33.93	24.58
5	0	27.3	64.24	369.82	475.48	**507.67**	465.84	427.65	328.38	51.26	26.18
6	0	13.52	43.37	74.14	189.49	**353.28**	269.74	222.73	176.51	136.81	31.57
7	0	59.43	107.44	247.16	364.02	**415.55**	306.18	186.7	102.24	60.49	7.95
8	0	84.78	117.77	172.69	236.02	295.73	**410.35**	228.01	110.57	52.97	5.98
9	0	57.49	111.52	229.15	**427.85**	324.46	254.91	134.78	70.88	30.27	3.83
10	0	88.45	171.12	271.78	292.41	**493.76**	257.12	178.61	32.13	22.41	9.48
11	0	150.12	248.33	**387.49**	287.88	205.68	116.93	84.62	52.07	39.03	7.76
12	0	55.25	97.38	150.56	195.01	239.85	**447.17**	249.51	136.64	18.06	3.76
13	0	29.15	53.08	266.48	370.12	**494.06**	437.54	401.3	348.4	57.42	1.79
14	0	122.45	274.88	319.25	359.93	375.2	**511.01**	369.51	115.62	48.48	16.53
15	0	50.32	96.22	195.03	**418.03**	322.83	277.34	228.37	144.21	19.79	16.16
16	0	77.94	94.49	189.88	212.98	284.36	293.39	**347.87**	134.29	48.22	18.99
Mean	0	79.33	144.84	252.50	332.69	367.13	333.21	252.02	137.24	47.32	13.62
S. D.	0	44.49	83.53	90.28	93.08	102.58	137.95	112.01	87.93	27.36	8.96
C.V.%	0	56.09	57.67	35.76	27.98	27.94	41.40	44.44	64.07	57.82	65.75

Vol. No.	(ng./ml.)		(hr.)		(ng. hr./ml.)		(ng. hr./ml.)		(hr.)		(hr.$^{-1}$)	
	A1	A2	A1	A2	A1	A2	A1	A2	A1	A2	A1	A2
1	478.6	462.0	2.5	2.5	2392.36	2564.97	2478.56	2720.35	4.14	4.92	0.167	0.141
2	406.6	517.3	3.0	3.0	1856.04	2412.56	1906.82	2473.14	4.04	3.97	0.171	0.175
3	311.2	375.5	2.0	2.0	1558.02	1851.25	1614.95	1923.25	4.55	4.56	0.152	0.152
4	496.3	633.3	4.0	4.0	3220.15	3804.22	3328.65	3957.01	4.27	4.31	0.162	0.161
5	471.6	507.7	3.0	3.0	3447.96	4064.05	3454.81	4233.12	2.53	4.48	0.274	0.155
6	495.5	353.3	4.0	3.0	3166.77	3118.10	3257.10	3406.26	4.06	6.33	0.170	0.110
7	362.3	415.6	2.5	3.0	1998.69	2460.35	2071.07	2503.74	4.10	3.78	0.169	0.183
8	360.9	410.4	3.0	4.0	1590.94	2462.94	1632.03	2492.13	3.98	3.38	0.174	0.205
9	320.6	427.9	2.5	2.5	1713.86	1871.22	1788.23	1888.93	4.26	3.20	0.163	0.216
10	316.4	493.8	3.0	3.0	1286.26	1968.38	1316.58	2021.85	3.90	3.91	0.178	0.177
11	615.3	387.5	2.0	2.0	2862.99	1709.77	2898.65	1757.01	3.44	4.22	0.202	0.164
12	621.1	447.2	4.0	4.0	4765.09	2237.71	4872.95	2253.34	3.99	2.88	0.174	0.241
13	324.5	494.1	3.0	3.0	2987.14	3784.06	3067.86	3790.45	4.46	2.48	0.155	0.280
14	327.3	511.0	4.0	4.0	2045.23	3307.60	2096.48	3406.16	3.93	4.13	0.176	0.168
15	591.0	418.0	2.0	2.5	2493.06	2255.40	2527.48	2355.48	3.51	4.29	0.197	0.161
16	602.8	347.9	4.0	6.0	4650.75	2610.40	4734.78	2741.86	3.82	4.80	0.181	0.144
N	16	16	16	16	16	16	16	16	16	16	16	16
Mean	443.86	450.14	3.03	3.22	2627.21	2655.18	2690.44	2745.26	3.94	4.10	0.18	0.18
SD	117.44	74.24	0.76	1.00	1046.19	744.94	1059.61	780.95	0.48	0.90	0.03	0.04
CV%	26.46	16.49	25.17	31.05	39.82	28.06	39.38	28.45	12.09	21.95	15.90	23.42

6 Mean Pharmacokinetic Parameters in 16 Volunteers with Reference and Test Preparation

harmacokinetic Parameters	Reference Preparation (A1)		Test Preparation (A2)	
C_{max} (ng./ml.)		443.86 ± 117.44		450.14 ± 74.24
t_{max} (hr.)	Mean ± S.D.	3.03 ± 0.76	Mean ± S.D.	3.22 ± 1.00
C 0-t (ng. hr./ml.)		2627.21 ± 1046.19		2655.18 ± 744.94
0-∞ (ng. hr. /ml.)		2690.44 ± 1059.61		2745.26 ± 780.95
k_{el} (hr.$^{-1}$)		0.179 ± 0.028		0.177 ± 0.041
$t_{1/2}$ (hr.)		3.937 ± 0.476		4.102 ± 0.900
e Bioavailability (%)	100 %		101.06%	

Blood Plasma Concentration Graph of Montelukast

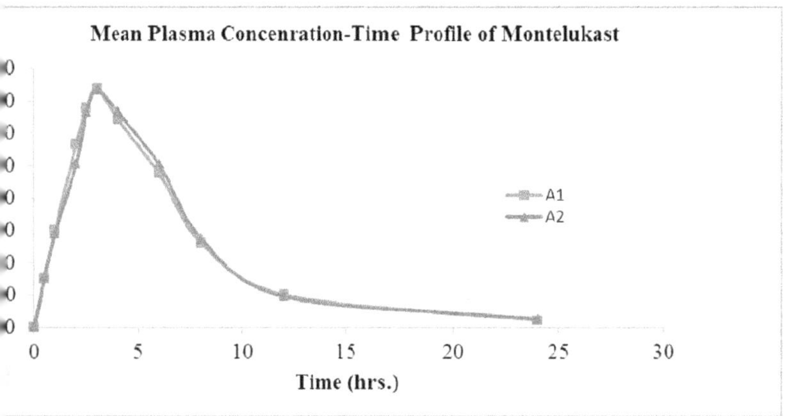

(A1- Reference Preparation; A2- Test Preparation)

...tive Pharmacokinetic Profile of Test and Reference Product
No. 1, 2 & 3)

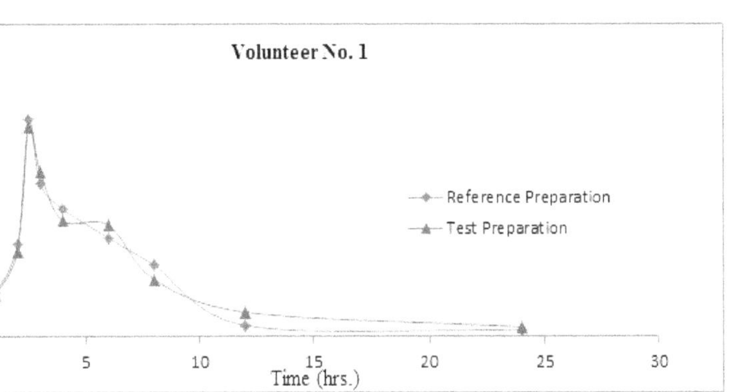

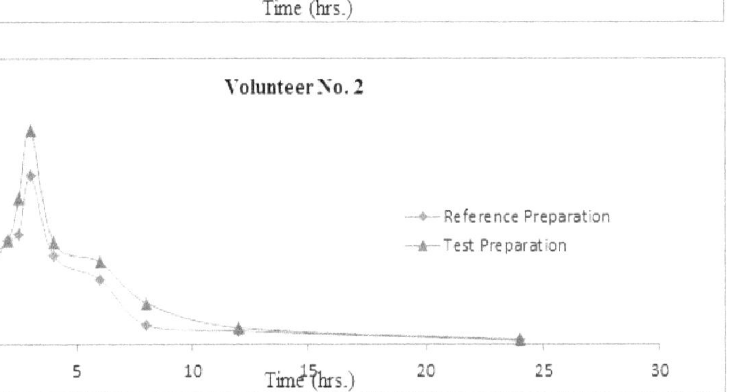

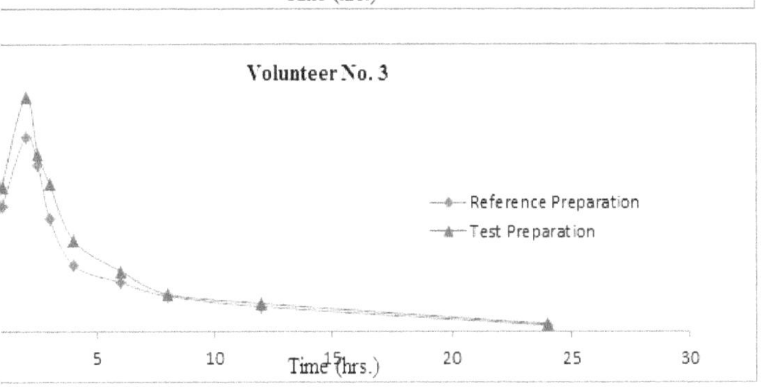

Bio-Analytical Method Development of Montelukast by LC-ESI-MS/MS

Introduction: A method has been developed for validation assay of single drug Montelukast 10 mg in human volunteer plasma using Propranolol as internal standard (IS).

Objectives: To describe the development of proposed method of analysis of single drug Montelukast 10 mg from plasma.

Method: Montelukast (CAS NO.-158966-92-8) which chemical formula $C_{35}H_{36}ClNO_3S$ is chemically (R, E)-2-(1-(1-(3-(2-(7-Chloroquinolin-2-yl) vinyl) phenyl)-3-(2-(2-hydroxypropan-2-yl) phenyl) propylthio) methyl) cyclopropyl) acetic acid which contain four consecutive rings. It is a leukotriene receptor antagonist used in the treatment of asthma and to relieve symtoms of seasonal allergies.

The exact and monoisotropic mass of Montelukast is 585.2104 (molecular wt. 586.2), H-bond donar count =2 and H-bond acceptor count =5 and rotable bond count=12. The P^{Ka} value of Montelukast 4.76 and 2.22 due to chloroquinolin ring and cyclopropyl respectively, so it is acidic drug. Due to significant difference in P^{Ka} value it was imperative to set optimum condition for plasma extraction, chromatography and mass detection for their simultaneous determination.

Propranolol used as internal standard (IS). For quantitation used positive polarity to achieve adequate response for their simultaneous analysis. Moreover positive ionization mode is selective and highly sensitive for compounds with low electron affinity. Thus positive ionization mode was selected to fragment the analyte and IS to obtain intense and consistent product ions. The protonated precursor ions $[M+H]^+$ at m/z 586.1(highest peak), 568.3(2nd peak), 570.1(3rd peak), were observed in Q1 MS for Montelukast and characteristic product ions or fragment ions found in Q3 MS were at m/z 422.2, 568.1, 440.3, 278.4. However the most stable and consistent fragment ion selected was m/z 422.2 for chloroquinolin ring.

For the internal standard The protonated precursor ions $[M+H]^+$ at m/z 260.2(highest peak) 254.9(2nd peak), 241.0(3rd peak), 239.0(4th peak))were observed in Q1 MS for propranolol and characteristic product ions or fragment ions found in Q3 MS were m/z 116.1, 183.0, 154.8, 129.0. However the most stable and consistent fragment ion selected was m/z 116.1 for naphthalene structure. The chromatographic elution of the analytes on *a* Phenomenex Kinetex 5μ C18 100A 50*3 mm column was initiated as a rapid, sensitive and rugged analytical method covering the dynamic linear range. The selection of mobile phase was crucial for synchronized determination of the drug having different pKa values. Thus, the pH of the mobile phase, buffer concentration, and choice and proportion of diluents were very which was important for chromatographic resolution with adequate response to achieve the desired sensitivity.

Structure	pKa Value	Nature	Fragment Ion (m/z)
Chloroquinolin	4.76	Acidic	422.2
Cyclopropyl	2.22	Acidic	586.1
Naphthalene	3.20	Acidic	116.1

Initially, acetonitrile/methanol with 5 mM ammonium acetate buffer (pH 6.5) gave response for montelukast and propranolol. However, the response was not reproducible. The signal was severely compromised at lower limit of quantitation (LLOQ) levels even after altering the concentration of buffer from 5 mM to 10 mM. Further, the chromatography was better with a higher response using a methanol-buffer as compared to an acetonitrile-buffer combination. Moreover, lowering the methanol content in the mobile phase resulted in an increase in the retention of montelukast and thereby the analysis time. Subsequent efforts were directed to optimize the pH of the mobile phase and the concentration of the buffer solution as they had significant impact on analyte retention, peak shape, and resolution. At pH above 5.0 the resolution of montelukast was unaffected, which further improved with increase in pH. Thus, to achieve greater reproducibility and better chromatography, high pH buffers were tried. Better reproducibility and peak shape were observed in 0.1% ammonia solution in methanol having, but the signal to noise ratio was not adequate at LLOQ level. Finally, a superior signal to noise ratio ($\geq$ 22) and baseline resolution was obtained for the analyte by replacing 10 Mm ammonium acetate buffer with 0.1% (v/v) ammonia solution together with Milli Q water having apparent pH 9.30 at a flow rate of 0.5000 mL/min.

There were no additional peaks due to endogenous plasma components as observed in one report when column was used even under MRM mode. The chromatographic elution time for montelukast & IS (propranolol) was 2.36 & 2.57 min, respectively, in a run time of 7.5 min. This analysis was done by gradation method in which 0.01 min to 0.70 min organic solvent 10% and then 0.70 min to 2.70 min organic solvent 90% and then from 2.70 min aqueous solvent 90% run upto 7.5 min for washing purpose.

Chemicals

Methanol	HPLC Grade
ACN	HPLC Grade
Water	HPLC Grade (From Milli Q water purification system)
Ammonia solution	AR Grade
Isopropyl Alcohol	AR Grade

Chromatographic Parameters

Component Name	Triple Quadrupole LC/MS/MS Mass Spectrometer
Component ID	API 2000
Manufacturer	AB Sciex Instruments
Model	029345/Q
Serial Number	B20510910
Column	PhenomenexKinetex 5μ C18 100 A 50*3 mm
Mobile Phase	A: 0.1% Ammonia sol^n in Milli Q water & mixed with 10 mM ammonium acetate
	B : 0.1% Ammonia solution in Methanol

Shimadzu LC Method Properties and Parameters

Shimadzu LC system Equilibration time	0.00 min
Shimadzu LC system Injection Volume	10.00 μl

Pumps	
Pump A Model	LC-20AD
Pump B Model	LC-20AD
Pumping Mode	Binary Flow
Total Flow	0.5000 mL/min.

System Controller	
Model	CBM-20A Lite
Power	On
Event 1	Off
Event 2	Off
Event 3	Off
Event 4	Off

Oven	
Model	CTO-10ASvp
Temperature Control	Disabled

Auto sampler	
Model	20AC
Rinsing Volume	200 μL
Needle Stroke	52 mm.
Rinsing Speed	35 μL/sec.
Sampling Speed	15.0 μL/sec.
Purge Time	25.0 min.
Rinse Dip Time	0 sec.
Cooler Enabled	Yes
Cooler Temperature	15°C
Control Vial Needle Stroke	52 mm

Time Program			
Time	Module	Events	Parameter
0.01	Pumps	Pump B Conc.	10
0.30	Pumps	Pump B Conc.	10
0.50	Pumps	Pump B Conc.	10
0.70	Pumps	Pump B Conc	10
1.00	Pumps	Pump B Conc.	90
1.50	Pumps	Pump B Conc.	90
2.50	Pumps	Pump B Conc	90
2.70	Pumps	Pump B Conc	90
3.00	Pumps	Pump B Conc	10
7.50	Controller	Stop	

Quantitation Information of Mass Spectrometry

Period 1 Experiment 1:	
Scan Type	MRM (MRM)
Scheduled MRM	No
Polarity	Positive
Scan Mode	N/A
Ion Source	Turbo Spray
Resolution Q1	Unit
Resolution Q3	Unit
Intensity Thres.:	0.00cps
Settling Time	0.0000msec
MR Pause	5.0070msec
MCA	No
Step Size	0.00Da

Montelukast (Analyte)	Q1 Mass (Da)	Q3 Mass (Da)	Dwell(msec)	Parameter	Start
	586.1	422.2	100.00	DP	20.0
				CE	35.0
				CXP	15.0

Propranolol (IS)	Q1 Mass (Da)	Q3 Mass (Da)	Dwell(msec)	Parameter	Start
	260.2	116.1	100.00	DP	30.0
				CE	31.0
				CXP	15.0

Parameters				
CUR	30.00		IS	5500.00
TEM	400.00		CAD	8.00
GS1	55.00		FP	400.00
GS2	45.00		EP	11.00

Keyed Text: File was created with the software version: Analyst 1.5

Internal Standard (IS)	
Drug Name	**Concentration**
Propranolol	1 µg/ml

Plasma Extraction Procedure: Plasma extraction was performed by **Protein precipitation technique,** 100 µl of plasma was taken and precipitated with 400 µl of MeCN containing 1000 ng/ml **Propranolol** (IS) and vortexed for 10 min, followed by Centrifugation for 10 mins at 12,000 rpm at 4°C. 300 µl supernatant was taken and transferred to auto sampler vials for injection.

Plasma Calibration Standards (ng/ml)

Montelukast: 10, 20, 40, 80, 160, 320, 640, 1280

QC Points

Montelukast:

	Montelukast:
LLOQ	10 ng/ml
LQC	30 ng/ml
MQC	480 ng/ml
HQC	960 ng/ml

Analytical and Bio-Analytical Results

Specificity & Selectivity: The specificity and selectivity of the assay is illustrated by the chromatograms of mobile phase run, and extract of blank plasma recorded for half an hour and an extract of a trial sample near the C_{max} for half an hour.

Sensitivity

> **Lower Limit of Detection (LLOD):**   1.8 ng/ml

> **Lower Limit of Quantification (LLOQ):** 10 ng/ml

Linearity of the Assay: The linearity of the calibration curve is determined by an unweighted least square regression analysis. A representative calibration curve of montelukast from human plasma is depicted in the linearity graph. The proposed assay is linear in the range of 10 ng/ml to 1280 ng/ml from plasma. (Refer: linearity detector response table). The representative calibration curve (code no. LIN I) is presented in linearity graph I.

Back calculated concentrations of the calibrate samples of the linearity and their statistical analysis is represented in LC-MS/MS data Table 1.

Table 1 Pre Study Linearity of Detector Response

Back Calculated Concentration of Calibrant Samples

Linearity	Concentration (ng/ml)							
	10	20	40	80	160	320	640	1280
LIN 1	9.78	20.67	41.48	76.6	161.28	337.08	641.91	1190.32
LIN 2	10.12	19.44	39.85	81.39	162.12	324.68	652.19	1223.48
LIN 3	10.88	16.70	39.39	75.04	167.09	348.15	658.90	1270.22
Average	10.26	18.94	40.24	77.68	163.50	336.64	651.00	1228.01
S.D	0.56	2.03	1.10	3.31	3.14	11.74	8.56	40.14
% C.V.	5.49	10.73	2.73	4.26	1.92	3.49	1.31	3.27
% Nominal	102.60	94.68	100.60	97.10	102.19	105.20	101.72	95.94

Plasma Calibration Curve of Montelukast

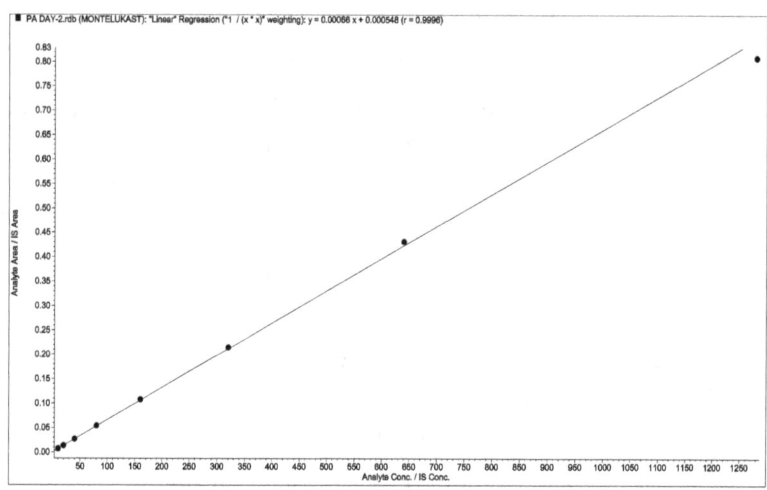

Table 2 LC-MS/MS Data

Pre Study Linearity of Detector Response

Linearity	Statistics		
Linearity Code	**Slope (m)**	**Intercept (c)**	**R square**
LIN 1	0.00066	0.00010	0.9987
LIN 2	0.00066	0.00055	0.9996
LIN 3	0.00068	0.00323	0.9951
Mean	0.0007		0.9978
S.D.	0.00001	Not Applicable	0.0024
C.V.%	1.8267		0.2386

Table 3 LC-MS/MS Data

Absolute Recovery (Area) of Montelukast from Plasma Samples

Inj. No.	Aqueous			In Plasma		
	QCL 30ng/ml	**QCM 480ng/ml**	**QCH 960ng/ml**	**QCL 30ng/ml**	**QCM 480ng/ml**	**QCH 960ng/ml**
1	3943.34	52141.92	104998.63	3814.94	52445.59	100538.17
2	3581.35	52464.78	99972.39	3546.52	53019.30	97224.47
3	3639.59	50798.99	96560.33	3722.95	50802.89	104257.76
4	3569.93	52638.91	105474.43	3282.16	49960.02	101402.25
5	3681.77	54074.49	101527.70	3620.47	54015.37	101886.49
Mean	**3683.20**	**52423.82**	**101706.70**	**3597.41**	**52048.63**	**101061.83**
	% Recovery			97.67	99.28	99.37

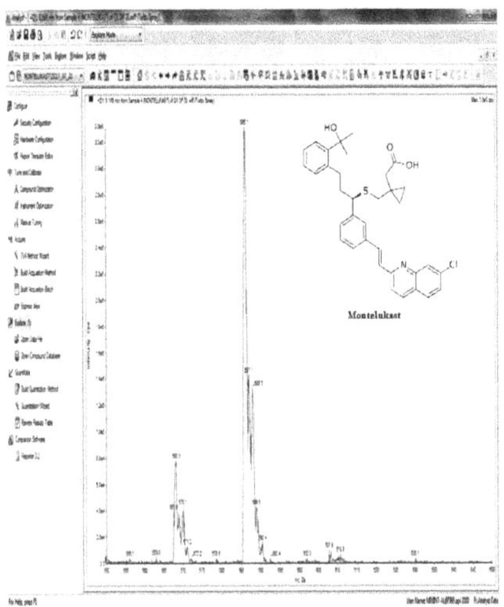

Figure 1 Montelukast Q-1 Scan

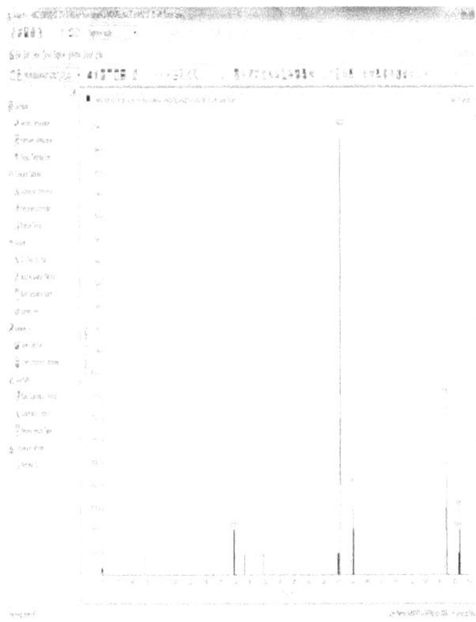

Figure 2 Montelukast Q-3 Scan

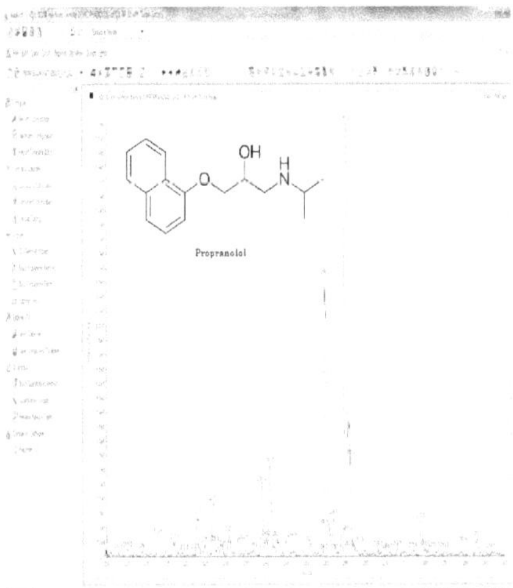

Figure 3 Propranolol Q-1 Scan

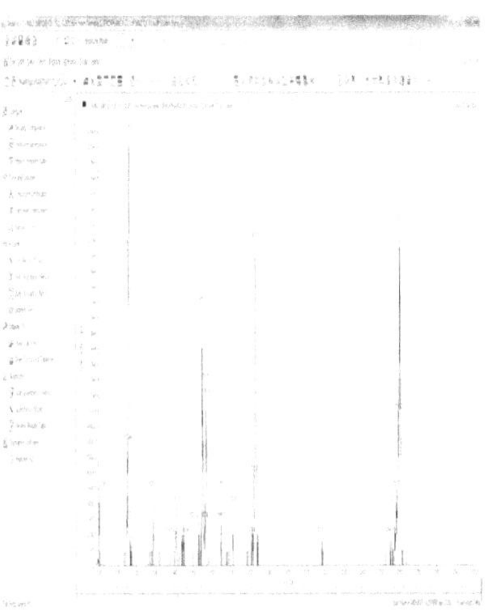

Figure 4 Propranolol Q-3 Scan

Recovery Experiment: The percentage recoveries were determined by measuring the peak areas of the drug from the prepared plasma low, medium and high quality control samples. The peak areas of the plasma low, medium and high quality control samples were compared to the absolute peak area of the unextracted standards containing the same concentrations of the montelukast. The results are presented in Table 3. Recovery after extraction was 97.67% - 99.37%.

Recovery of Internal Standard: The % Recoveries were determined by measuring the peak areas of the IS from the prepared plasma low, medium, high quality control samples. The peak areas of the plasma Low, Medium and high quality control samples were compared to the absolute peak area of the unextracted standard containing the same concentrations of the IS. Recovery after extraction was 91.18% to 97.28% for montelukast.

Table 3 A LC-MS/MS Data
Absolute Recovery (Area) of Internal Standard (Propranolol)
from Plasma Samples

Inj. No.	Aqueous			In Plasma		
	QCL 30 ng/ml	QCM 480 ng/ml	QCH 960 ng/ml	QCL 30 ng/ml	QCM 480 ng/ml	QCH 960 ng/ml
1	434386.39	418165.58	377934.72	438220.69	394691.92	401877.47
2	409604.83	431399.70	436282.15	418729.16	412427.03	405436.61
3	411453.64	399836.67	404313.31	414331.43	327531.07	445902.66
4	411712.45	439747.58	473985.29	367083.69	403751.77	432130.51
5	404655.84	447084.08	406258.36	377100.95	409422.66	343860.84
Mean	414362.63	427246.72	419754.77	403093.18	389564.89	405841.62
	% Recovery			97.28	91.18	96.69

Precision and Accuracy: Between–run precision and accuracy are determined from the low, medium and high QC samples (QCL, QCM, and QCH). A total of 5 replicates of each QC concentration were assayed on day 1 and a total of 5 replicates each QC concentration were assayed on day 2 and 3. The QC samples concentrations were determined from three different calibration curves that were assayed with QC samples. Precision as expressed as percent variation (%CV), while accuracy is measured as the percent nominal (% nominal) (LC-MS/MS Data Table 4). Between–run precision values (%CV) ranged from **5.041%** to **6.849%**. Between – run accuracy values (% nominal) were **96.45%** for LLOQ, **94.82%** for low QC (QCL), **94.23%** for medium QC (QCM) and **93.44%** for high QC (QCH) samples.

Within-run precision and accuracy are determined from a total of 5 replicates of each QC concentration. The low, medium and high QC samples (QCL, QCM, and QCH) assayed on day 1. The QC samples concentrations were determined from calibration curves LIN1. Precision as expressed as percent variation (%CV), while accuracy is measured as the percent nominal (LC-MS/MS Data Table 5). Within-run precision values (%CV) ranged from **1.809%** to **6.758%**. Within-run accuracy values (% nominal) were **94.78%** for LLOQ, **91.76%** for low QC (QCL), **96.52%** for medium QC (QCM) and **90.94%** for high QC (QCH) samples.

Table 4 LC-MS/MS Data
Precision and Accuracy (Between Run)

Linearity Code	LLOQ 10 ng/ml	QCL 30 ng/ml	QCM 480 ng/ml	QCH 960 ng/ml
LIN 1	10.16	30.00	453.65	838.65
LIN 1	9.38	26.99	432.16	870.49
LIN 1	9.86	28.68	423.85	877.49
LIN 1	10.05	27.44	434.96	888.16
LIN 1	10.32	28.94	441.51	879.03
LIN 2	10.54	28.68	486.50	876.40
LIN 2	9.02	26.81	473.03	849.57
LIN 2	9.31	26.23	448.04	881.48
LIN 2	8.96	27.77	453.27	891.07
LIN 2	9.56	28.15	455.71	866.80
LIN 3	8.97	25.53	445.44	903.96
LIN 3	8.45	29.17	443.07	943.25
LIN 3	9.23	31.01	435.99	865.59
LIN 3	10.57	30.27	512.00	1036.74
LIN 3	10.29	31.02	445.17	987.14
Mean	**9.645**	**28.446**	**452.290**	**897.055**
S.D.	**0.661**	**1.682**	**22.799**	**53.169**
C.V.%	**6.849**	**5.911**	**5.041**	**5.927**
Absolute %bias (%)	**96.45**	**94.82**	**94.23**	**93.44**

Table 5 LC-MS/MS Data
Precision and Accuracy (Within Run)

Inj. No.	Montelukast			
	LLOQ 10 ng/ml	QCL 30 ng/ml	QCM 480 ng/ml	QCH 960 ng/ml
1	10.54	28.68	486.50	876.40
2	9.02	26.81	473.03	849.57
3	9.31	26.23	448.04	881.48

Table 5 contd....

4	8.96	27.77	453.27	891.07
5	9.56	28.15	455.71	866.80
Mean	9.478	27.528	463.310	873.064
S.D.	0.640	0.997	16.000	15.791
C.V.%	6.758	3.620	3.453	1.809
Absolute percent bias (%)	**94.78**	**91.76**	**96.52**	**90.94**

Table 6 LC-MS/MS Data
Freeze Thaw Recovery

Inj. No.	Freeze thawed			After Three Cycles		
	QCL 30ng/ml	**QCM 480ng/ml**	**QCH 960ng/ml**	**QCL 30ng/ml**	**QCM 480ng/ml**	**QCH 960ng/ml**
1	25.53	445.44	903.96	29.76	467.33	874.5
2	29.17	443.07	943.25	27.92	434.04	876.19
3	31.01	435.99	865.59	26.55	449.18	893.37
4	30.27	512.00	1036.74	29.02	439.9	859.99
5	31.02	445.17	987.14	26.80	426.01	879.73
Mean	**29.40**	**456.33**	**947.34**	**28.01**	**443.29**	**876.76**
	% Stability			**95.27**	**97.14**	**92.55**

Freeze Thaw Recovery: The stability of low, medium and high quality control samples were determined after three freeze thaw cycles comparing against freshly thawed samples of the same concentration. The stability of montelukast ranges between 92.55% - 97.14% after three cycles.

Short Term Stability: The stability of low, medium and high quality control samples were determined after keeping the samples on the bench top for 24 hrs and comparing against fresh samples of the same concentration. The short term stability (Table 7) of montelukast ranges between 94.76% to 96.44% after three cycles.

Table 7 LC-MS/MS Data
Short Term Stability (24 hrs)

Montelukast				After 24 Hrs.		
	QCL 30ng/ml	**QCM 480ng/ml**	**QCH 960ng/ml**	**QCL 30ng/ml**	**QCM 480ng/ml**	**QCH 960ng/ml**
1	25.53	445.44	903.96	29.44	461.95	908.23
2	29.17	443.07	943.25	27.69	429.97	947.62
3	31.01	435.99	865.59	27.37	434.69	920.22
4	30.27	512.00	1036.74	27.59	439.24	892.58
5	31.02	445.17	987.14	27.2	434.2	899.2
Mean	**29.40**	**456.33**	**947.34**	**27.86**	**440.01**	**913.57**
	% Stability			**94.76**	**96.42**	**96.44**

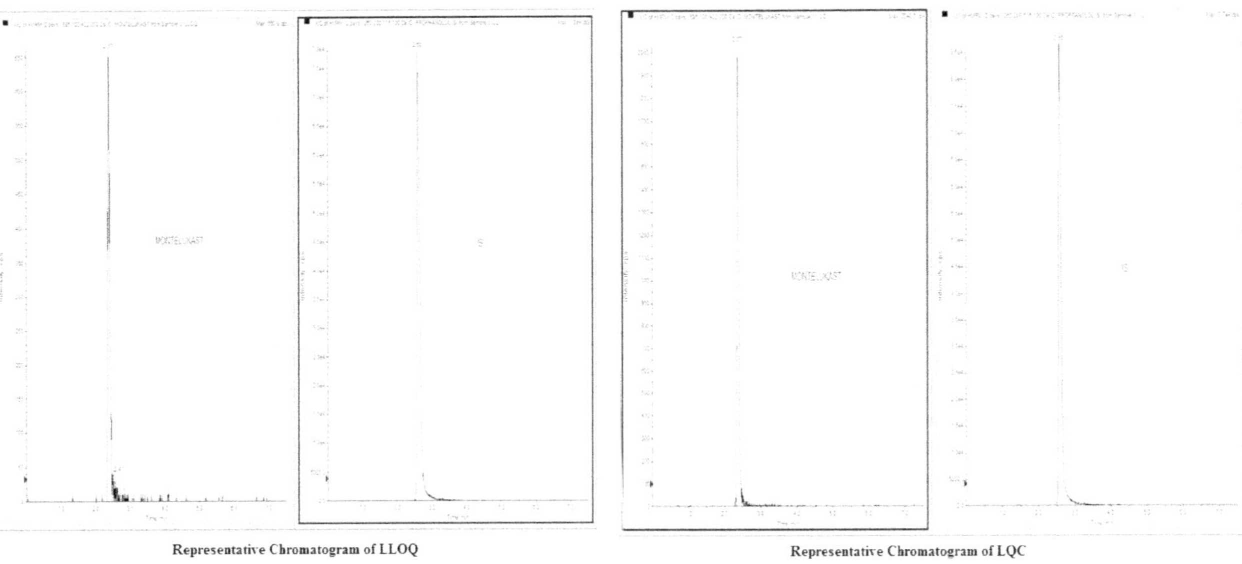

Representative Chromatogram of LLOQ

Representative Chromatogram of LQC

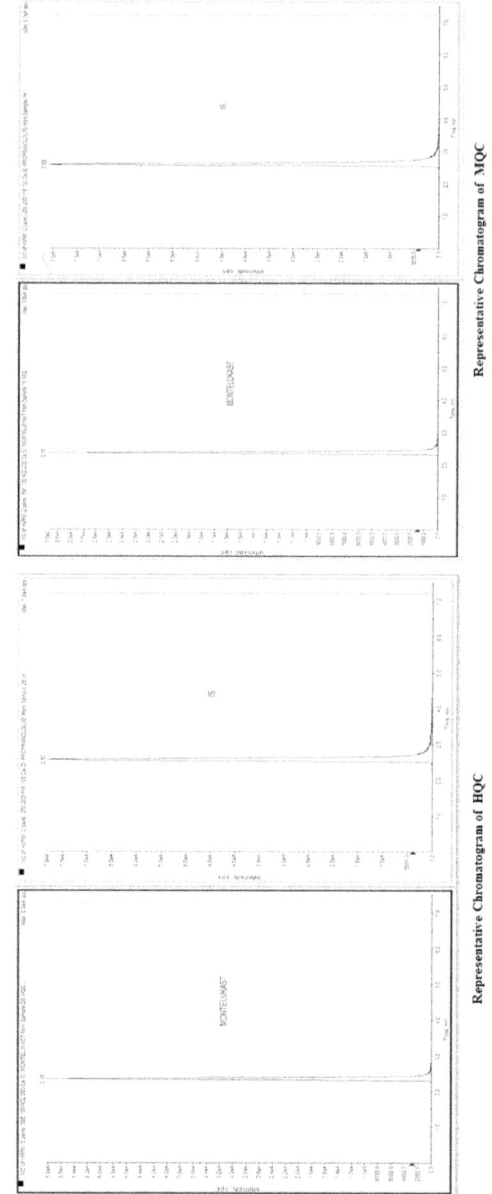

Representative Chromatogram of MQC

Representative Chromatogram of HQC

Table 8 LC-MS/MS Data
Long Term Stability (15 days)

Montelukast	QCL 30ng/ml	QCM 480ng/ml	QCH 960ng/ml	After 15 days in freezer		
				QCL 30ng/ml	QCM 480ng/ml	QCH 960ng/ml
1	25.53	445.44	903.96	30.62	479.03	856.3
2	29.17	443.07	943.25	26.87	429.2	864.48
3	31.01	435.99	865.59	27.62	435.72	878.47
4	30.27	512.00	1036.74	27.67	426.88	854.36
5	31.02	445.17	987.14	26.82	420.88	835.99
Mean	**29.40**	**456.33**	**947.34**	**27.92**	**438.34**	**857.92**
	% Stability			**94.97**	**96.06**	**90.56**

Long Term Stability: The long term stability (Table 8) of low and high quality control samples were determined by comparing bench top against samples analyzed after 15 days. The short term stability of montelukast was resulted in 90.56% to 96.06% for QCL and QCH respectively.

Auto Sampler Stability: The auto sampler stability (Table 9) of low and high quality control samples were determined by comparing bench top against samples kept in auto sampler for 24 hrs. The auto sampler stability of montelukast was resulted in 92.03% to 95.95% for QCL and QCH respectively.

Table 9 LC-MS/MS Data
Auto Sampler Stability

Montelukast	QCL 30ng/ml	QCM 480ng/ml	QCH 960ng/ml	After 24hrs in Auto sampler		
				QCL 30ng/ml	QCM 480ng/ml	QCH 960ng/ml
1	25.53	445.44	903.96	31.21	454.3	829.74
2	29.17	443.07	943.25	26.07	419.8	902.79
3	31.01	435.99	865.59	26.62	411.75	936.96
4	30.27	512.00	1036.74	25.88	451.83	826.41
5	31.02	445.17	987.14	25.70	451.55	863.42
Mean	**29.40**	**456.33**	**947.34**	**27.10**	**437.85**	**871.86**
	% Stability			**92.16**	**95.95**	**92.03**

Matrix Effect: The Matrix Effect of Internal Standard (Propranolol) ranges between 90.97% - 93.39% (Table 10) and for montelukast, it ranges between 90.58% to 95.79% after three cycles.

Table 10 LC-MS/MS Data

Matrix Effect (Area) of Inernal Standard (Propranolol)

Sample	Extracted Blank Plasma	Aqueous	Matrix Effect %	Matrix Factor
LQC1	316379.91	360679.81	87.72	0.88
LQC2	279638.72	304441.12	91.85	0.92
LQC3	314479.48	353772.45	88.89	0.89
LQC4	293070.59	328498.56	89.22	0.89
LQC5	313403.65	322607.73	97.15	0.97
Mean	**303394.47**	**333999.93**	**90.97**	**0.91**
S.D.	**16298.78**	**23111.36**	**3.77**	**0.04**
C.V.%	**5.37**	**6.92**	**4.15**	**4.04**
MQC1	402995.99	410768.37	98.11	0.98
MQC2	430560.83	476059.80	90.44	0.90
MQC3	432811.49	443867.09	97.51	0.97
MQC4	430648.33	475541.21	90.56	0.90
MQC5	452565.11	501068.82	90.32	0.90
Mean	**429916.35**	**461461.06**	**93.39**	**0.93**
S.D.	**17656.48**	**34854.86**	**4.04**	**0.04**
C.V.%	**4.11**	**7.55**	**4.33**	**4.43**
HQC1	314149.76	357132.34	87.96	0.88
HQC2	379918.11	382446.88	99.34	0.99
HQC3	331562.08	376665.41	88.03	0.88
HQC4	281668.04	303444.00	92.82	0.93
HQC5	295063.65	300713.58	98.12	0.98
Mean	**320472.33**	**344080.44**	**93.25**	**0.93**
S.D.	**38236.54**	**39484.56**	**5.39**	**0.05**
C.V.%	**11.93**	**11.48**	**5.78**	**5.65**

Table 10 A LC-MS/MS Data

Matrix Effect (Area) of Analyte (Montelukast)

Sample	Extracted Blank Plasma	Aqueous	Matrix Effect %	Matrix Factor
LQC1	3294.93	3295.20	99.99	0.99
LQC2	2910.12	2937.12	99.08	0.99
LQC3	2749.62	3011.01	91.32	0.91
LQC4	2801.1	2950.06	94.95	0.95
LQC5	2712.93	2898.39	93.60	0.94
Mean	**2893.74**	**3018.36**	**95.79**	**0.96**
S.D.	**236.26**	**159.96**	**3.67**	**0.03**
C.V.%	**8.16**	**5.30**	**3.83**	**3.59**
MQC1	51179.72	58010.57	88.22	0.88
MQC2	53606.58	54162.27	98.97	0.99
MQC3	51973.73	59344.22	87.58	0.88
MQC4	50587.11	55355.38	91.39	0.91
MQC5	53531.09	61706.87	86.75	0.87
Mean	**52175.65**	**57715.86**	**90.58**	**0.91**
S.D.	**1363.90**	**3035.89**	**5.01**	**0.05**
C.V.%	**2.61**	**5.26**	**5.53**	**5.44**
HQC1	91915.87	102452.30	89.72	0.90
HQC2	93019.35	100070.92	92.95	0.93
HQC3	84294.86	85581.06	98.50	0.98
HQC4	84647.13	85197.34	99.35	0.99
HQC5	79843.11	84787.20	94.17	0.94
Mean	**86744.06**	**91617.76**	**94.94**	**0.95**
S.D.	**5571.03**	**8848.21**	**4.00**	**0.04**
C.V.%	**6.42**	**9.66**	**4.21**	**3.90**

Conclusion

This method was found to be simple, reproducible, sensitive, and specific for the determination of montelukast from plasma. Hence, this method can be applied to study the pharmacokinetic parameters of montelukast.

VALIDATION OF A LIQUID CHROMATOGRAPHY MASS SPECTROMETRY METHOD FOR THE DETERMINATION OF MONTELUKAST IN PLASMA

Method Validation Protocol
MV Protocol Number: MVP- 01/17/393
Status: Final Version: 1.0
Date: 22.01.17

Study Protocol Number: 01/17/393
Status: Final Version: 1.0
Date: 22.01.17

Protocol Prepared by:

....

Protocol Approved by:

....

Sponsor:

....

....

Name of CRO & Address

....

....

....

1.0   Authentication

1.1   Bioanalytical Declaration

We, the undersigned, authenticate that we have reviewed this protocol thoroughly and critically and have evaluated the same.

Head – Bio-Analytical

(Name, Signature & Date)

Technical Advisor/ Director

(Name, Signature & Date)

Approval

I, the undersigned approve that I have thoroughly reviewed this protocol for anomalies and compliance and critically evaluated the scientific validity of the statements in this protocol and to the best of my knowledge and judgment this protocol is scientifically valid.

Head, Quality Assurance (QA)

(Name, Signature & Date)

2.0   Method Validation Schedule

Schedule	Timelines
Method Validation	
Preparation of Method validation Report	
Review of Method validation Report by Head- BA	
QA Review	

MV Report of Montelukast (xx/xx/xxx)

3.0   List of Abbreviations

AR	:	Analytical Reagent
BA	:	Bio-analytical
CAL	:	Calibration Standard
g	:	Gram
GR	:	General Reagent Grade
HPLC	:	High Performance Liquid Chromatography
HQC	:	High Quality Control
IS	:	Internal Standard
LQC	:	Lower Quality Control
LR	:	Laboratory Reagent Grade
M	:	Method
mg	:	Milligram
mL	:	Milliliter
MQC	:	Middle Quality Control
ng	:	Nanogram
No.	:	Number
P&A	:	Precision and Accuracy
QA	:	Quality Assurance
QC	:	Quality Control
RA	:	Research Associate
SOP	:	Standard Operating Procedure
TBME	:	Tert-Butyl Methyl Ether

4.0   Description of Materials

Test Article: Refer Annexure I for the certificate of analysis

Working Standard	Montelukast
Batch No	MTN(M)/15066A
Expiry	Oct,2018
Purity	99.74%
Storage	Room Temperature (RT)
Mol. Wt.	586.184 g/mol
Source	Melody HealthCare

Internal Standard: Refer Annexure II for the certificate of analysis

Working Standard	Propanolol
Batch No	SBP-PRL-032
Expiry	20/07/2018
Purity	97%
Storage	Refrigerator (2 to 8°C)
Mol. Wt.	295.80 g/mol
Source	Subham Biopharma

5.0   Objective

To describe the process as well as validate a bio analytical method for estimation of Montelukast in Human plasma using Propranolol as an internal standard (IS).

6.0   Scope

This procedure is applicable for the analysis of Montelukast in human plasma.

7.0   Study Personnel Name and Roles

S.no	Personnel name	Roles
1.		Review of Final protocols
2.	Members of Analytical Team	Bulk spiking, Sample processing, Instrument operation
3.		Sample processing

8.0 Procedure

8.1 Experimental

8.1.1 Chemical, Reagents and Matrix

Chemical	Reagents	Matrix
Montelukast (Working Standard)	Methanol & Dimethyl Sulfoxide (DMSO)	Blank Human Plasma
Propranolol (Internal Standard)		
Ammonia Solution (AR Grade) & Ammonium Acetate (AR Grade)		
Milli Q Water (HPLC Grade)		

8.1.2 Equipment

Equipment	Make	Serial Number
HPLC pump	Shimadzu LC20AD	L20104717592
HPLC Autosampler	Shimadzu SIL20AC HT	L20354701578
Triple Quadrupole Mass Spectrometer API 2000	AB Sciex Instruments	B20510910
Deep Freezer (-20°C)	Celfrost	091131273
Centrifuge	REMI	CPLC-1503
pH meter	Sartorius	PB-11
Top loading balance	Sartorious	17505932

8.2 Preparation of Solutions

8.2.1 Preparation of Mobile Phase A

10 mm Ammonium Acetate in water with 0.1% Ammonia Solution. Add 0.7708 mg of ammonium acetate in 1000 mL of Milli Q Grade Water in a 1000 mL reagent bottle and add 1 mL of ammonia solution. Sonicate for 5 minutes. Use this solution within 3 days from the date of preparation. Provide a batch number.

8.2.2 Preparation of Mobile phase B

0.1% Ammonia Solution in Methanol. Add 1 ml of ammonia solution in 1000 mL of Methanol. Filtered and sonicate for 5 minutes. Use this solution within 3 days from the date of preparation. Provide a batch number.

8.3   Preparation of Stock Solution

8.3.1 Montelukast Stock Solution (W/V)

Weigh about 10 mg of montelukast and dissolve in 10 mL DMSO. Mix well and sonicate. Correct the above final concentration for Montelukast accounting its potency and the actual amount weighed. This is stock solution. Provide a batch number and complete the 'Stock Weighing and Solution Preparation Form'. Store in refrigerator at 2-8°C.

8.3.2 Propanolol (ISTD) Stock Solution (W/V)

Weigh about 10 mg of propanolol and dissolve in 10 mL DMSO. Correct the above final concentration for propanolol accounting for its potency and the actual amount weighed. Provide a batch number and complete the 'Stock Weighing and Solution Preparation. Store in a refrigerator at 2-8°C.

8.4.1.4 Preparation of Intermediate Concentration

Table A Preparation of Intermediate Concentration

Stock Conc. (µg /mL)	Stock Aliquot (µL)	Diluent Added (µL)	Final Volume (mL)	Final Conc. (µg/mL)
1000	100	900	1	100

Table B Preparation of Intermediate Concentration

Stock Conc. (µg /mL)	Stock Aliquot (µL)	Diluent Added (µL)	Final Volume (mL)	Final Conc. (µg/mL)
100	100	900	1	10

Table C Preparation of Intermediate Concentration

Stock Conc. (µg /mL)	Stock Aliquot (µL)	Diluent Added (µL)	Final Volume (mL)	Final Conc. (µg/mL)
10	100	900	1	1

Table D Preparation of Intermediate Concentration

Stock Conc. (µg /mL)	Stock Aliquot (µL)	Diluent Added (µL)	Final Volume (mL)	Final Conc. (µg/mL)
1	100	900	1	100

8.4.1.5 Preparation of Stock Dilutions

Prepare stock dilutions of Montelukast in the concentration of 1280 ng/mL to 10 ng/mL using intermediate starting concentration 1 mg/mL.

Table E Preparation of Montelukast Stock Dilutions

Stock Conc. (ng/mL)	Stock volume taken (µL)	Solvent added (µL)	Final Conc. (ng/mL)
10000	2560	7440	2560
10000	1280	8720	1280
1000	640	360	640
1000	320	680	320
1000	160	840	160
100	800	200	80
100	400	600	40
100	200	800	20

8.4.1.4 Drug spiking in blank Human plasma for Calibration Curve

Transfer 500 µl of each of the corresponding concentrations of the above described stock dilutions of Montelukast into 500 µl blank Human plasma to achieve calibration conc. points given below.

Table F Preparation of Montelukast Calibration Solution in Spiked Plasma

Stock Concentrations of Montelukast (µg/mL)	Montelukast Concentration in spiked plasma (µg/mL)	Spiked plasma Concentration ID
2560	1280	CC8
1280	640	CC7
640	320	CC6
320	160	CC5
160	80	CC4
80	40	CC3
40	20	CC2
20	10	CC1

Concentrations in plasma represent uncorrected concentrations. True concentrations may vary as per potency and the actual amount weighed. Pipette 0.180 mL blank human plasma aliquot of each calibration spiked standard into polypropylene-capped tubes and freeze at -20°C until analysis.

8.4.2 Quality Control (QC) Samples

8.4.2.1 Preparation of Stock Dilutions

Prepare QC stock dilutions of Montelukast in a concentration using diluents as described in the Table G below.

Table G Preparation of Quality Control Stock Dilution

Stock Conc. Montelukast (ng/mL)	Stock Aliquot (µL)	Diluent Added (µL)	Final Volume (mL)	Final Conc. (ng/mL)
10000	1920	8080	1	1920
1000	960	40	1	960
100	60	40	1	60

8.4.2.2 Spiking of Plasma for Quality Control Samples

Transfer 500 µl of each of the corresponding concentrations of the above described stock dilutions into 500 µl blank Human plasma to achieve HQC, MQC and LQC respectively.

Table H Preparation of Montelukast QC Concentration in Spiked Plasma

Stock Conc. (µg/mL)	Final Conc. in spiked plasma (ng/mL)	Spiked Plasma Conc. ID
1920	960	HQC
960	480	MQC
60	30	LQC

Concentrations in plasma represent uncorrected concentrations. True concentrations may vary as per potency and the actual amount weighed. Pipette 100 µL aliquot of each quality control samples into polypropylene-capped tubes and freeze at -20°C until analysis.

8.5   Bio Analytical Method

8.5.1 Sample Preparation

Withdraw the spiked human plasma samples from the deep freezer and allow them to thaw at room temperature

Add 100 µL of aliquot and 400 µL internal standard (Propranolol – 5µg/mL) into 2 mL centrifuge tubes

Vortex for 10 minutes

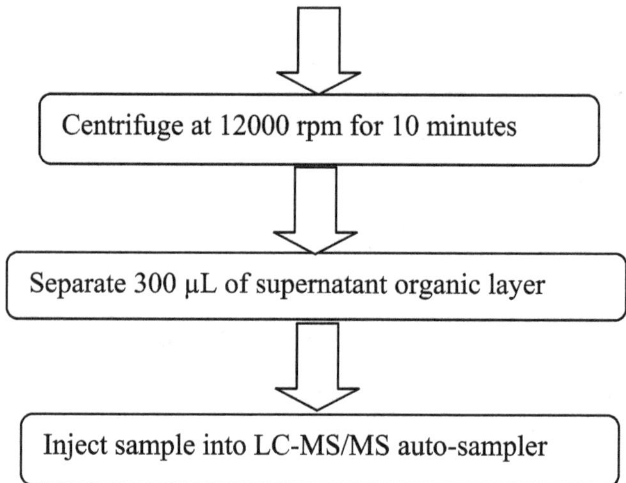

8.5.2   Chromatographic Conditions

Column	Phenomenex Kinetex C18; 50 x 3 mm , Particle Size- 5 µm
Mobile Phase	**A :** H_2O with 10 mM Ammonium Acetate with 0.1% Ammonia Solution **B :** MeOH with 0.1% Ammonia Solution
Flow rate	0.5 mL/min.
Injection volume	5.00 µL
Total run time(min)	4.0 min.
Auto sampler Temperature	10 -15°C
Retention Time (min)	Montelukast: 2.47 Propranolol (IS): 2.67

The mobile phase and the flow rate may be modified to optimize the chromatographic response. The retention times listed should not be considered as method specifications but as assay method parameters.

8.5.3 Multiple Reaction Monitoring (MRM) Conditions

Compound	Q1	Q3	Dwell Time	DP	CE	CXP
Montelukast	586.1	422.2	100.00	20.0	35.0	15.0
Propranolol (IS)	260.2	116.1	100.00	30.0	31.0	15.0
DP = Declustering Potential; CE = Collision Energy; CXP = Collision Cell Exit Potential						

9.0 Validation Parameters

9.1 Selectivity

A minimum of six matrix lots will be used and screened for selectivity out of which one is heamolytic and one is lipemic. From each lot of matrix, a blank and LLOQ sample is spiked and processed as per the method procedure. The processed samples were injected and analyzed. The interference in the blank matrix will be evaluated by comparing the response at the retention time of analyte and internal standard against the response of analyte and internal standard in the extracted LLOQ samples.

Acceptance Criteria

- Response of the interfering peak at the retention time of analyte should be ≤20% of mean response of analyte(s) in LLOQ concentration.

- For internal standard, the response of the interfering peak at the RT of IS should be ≤5% of mean response of IS in LLOQ sample.

9.2 Back Calculated Concentrations for Calibration Curve Standards

Back calculations will be made from the calibration curves to determine concentrations of calibration standards (Table B) of the analyte. Any one of LLOQ and ULOQ (submitted in duplicate) should compulsorily pass and no two consequent points should fail. All the calibration curve points, HQC, MQC and LQC samples should be within ±15% of the specified concentrations, except for the LLOQ within ±20%. 75% of the calibration standards should be within the acceptance range including the lowest and highest calibration standard.

While considering the individual QC level a minimum of 50% should be within acceptance range. Overall a minimum of 67% of the QC's in the P & A batch should be within acceptance range. Remaining 33% of the QC samples (not all the replicates at the same concentration) may be above 15% provided the mean accuracy values are within the acceptance range. % CV should be within ±15% at HQC, MQC, LQC and ±20% levels.

9.3 Precision and Accuracy

9.3.1 Within–Batch Accuracy and Precision

The within–batch accuracy and precision shall be assessed by the repeated analysis of blood samples containing different concentrations on three P&A batches using 2 analysts on separate occasions. A single run consists of a calibration curve plus 6 replicates of the LQC, MQC and

HQC samples in singlets. In Calibration curve LLOQ and ULOQ samples alone are run in duplicates.

9.3.2 Between-Batch Accuracy and Precision

The between–batch accuracy and precision shall be assessed by the repeated analysis of precision and accuracy batches containing different concentrations of drug on two consecutive days. Two precision and accuracy batches shall be carried out on a single day and the third batch on the other day. A single run consists of a calibration curve plus 6 replicates of the LQC, MQC and HQC in singlets. In Calibration curve LLOQ and ULOQ samples alone are run in duplicates.

9.3.3 Run Acceptance Criteria

Any one of LLOQ and ULOQ should compulsorily pass and no two consequent points should fail. All the calibration curve points, HQC, MQC and LQC samples should be within ±15% of the specified concentrations, except for the LLOQ within ±20%. While considering the individual QC level a minimum of 50% should be within acceptance range. Overall a minimum of 67% of the QC's in the P & A batch should be within acceptance range. Remaining 33% of the QC samples (not all the replicates at the same concentration) may be above 15% provided the mean accuracy values are within the acceptance range. % CV is within ±15% at HQC, MQC, LQC and ±20% LLOQ Quality Control levels.

9.4   Recovery

Six replicates of extracted HQC, MQC and LQC are prepared as per the method procedure. Freshly prepared aqueous QC samples based on recovery along with the extracted QC samples are injected. The mean peak area response of the extracted samples is compared with the mean peak area response of the aqueous samples. The mean of % recovery, standard deviation and %CV are calculated for each level and the global mean % recovery of analyte and internal standards are calculated. % Recovery for analyte(s) and IS (s) should not be more than 115% and % CV of area at different concentrations (*i.e.,* HQC, MQC and LQC) should be <15%. % CV of Global Recovery should be ±20%.

9.5   Stock Solution Stability

9.5.1 Short-term Stock Solution Stability

Short term stock solution stability for the analyte and the internal standard shall be assessed after 6 hours at room temperature along with freshly prepared stock solution at middle level quality control concentration. The mean peak response of the "0" hour and "n" hour stock solution(s) should be within the range of 85- 115%.

9.5.2 Long-term Stock Solution Stability

Long term stock solution stability for the analyte and the internal standard shall be assessed for a minimum of 3 days or for the prescribed time at 2 to 8°C along with freshly prepared stock solution at middle level quality control concentration. The mean peak response of "0" hr and "n" hr stock solution(s) should be within the range of 85- 115%.

9.6   Stability of Drug in Matrix

9.6.1 Freeze Thaw Stability

A calibration curve shall be processed along with 6 replicates of stability samples at low and high QC levels which shall be subjected to four freeze thaw cycles. In first cycle sample shall be frozen at -80°C for 24 hrs, then it shall be thawed to room temperature until it gets completely thawed. The second cycle and the subsequent cycles shall be further frozen at -80°C for minimum 12 hrs & thawed to room temperature. After 4th cycle samples shall be analyzed in a single run. Mean concentration obtained for stability QC samples should be 85-115% of nominal concentration of freshly prepared QC samples. % CV should be within ±15%.

9.6.2 Auto Sampler Stability

Auto sampler stability can be defined as on-instrument/ auto-sampler stability of the processed sample at injector or auto-sampler temperature.

9.7   Matrix Effect

Six different lots of blood shall be processed in duplicates (without spiking analyte and internal standard) as per the extraction procedure and before reconstitution step, the aqueous HQC and LQC samples are spiked with internal standard and analyzed. Aqueous samples shall be prepared based on recovery for both analyte and internal standard at HQC and LQC levels and injected along with the post spiked samples and analyzed to determine the effect of matrix with the analyte or the internal standard. Matrix effect should be within ±15% and 75% of lots used should pass the matrix effect.

10.0 Data Processing

Acquire chromatograms using the computer-based software supplied by AB Sciex Instruments Analyst 1.6.3 by peak area ratio. Determine the standard curve fitting the concentration and response relationship using linear $1/x^2$ weighing and statistical tests for goodness of fit.

$$y = mx+c$$

Where x = concentration of Montelukast

y = peak area ratio of Montelukast

c = y axis intercept of the calibration curve

11.0 Method Validation Protocol Structure

The method validation shall be performed as per Guidelines for Bioavailability & Bioequivalence Studies published by Central Drugs Standard Control Organization in March 2005.

12.0 Quality Control Role

QC staff will check the Method validation raw data, results, log book entries and related documentation as follows:

- Raw data
- Log books and the data
- Weighing printout
- Documentation of any SOP / protocol deviation.
- Analytical run sequence
- Results table and chromatograms

13.0 Quality Assurance Role

QA staff shall monitor/ inspect and audit the following activities:

- Stock solution preparation.
- Bulk spiking of CCs and QCs
- Forms issue and control
- Inspection during the method validation   experiments
- Checking and auditing of raw data entries and assuring that the results are transcribed correctly in the method validation protocol
- QA authentication of Method validation protocol

14.0 Record Keeping

The method validation raw data and chromatograms are compiled and after the approval of QA the files (hard copy, soft copy) are maintained in the archive for a period of 15 years from the date of signing of the protocol.

15.0 Method Validation Protocol Deviations

Concentrations reflected in the protocol are suggested ranges for Calibration Curve and Quality control samples may be altered to specific needs of the study design. The concentrations should be within the range given in the method validation protocol. The chromatographic parameters and instrumentation parameters may also be optimized to get the specific response for the analytes and internal standard. Apart from this any other deviations from the method validation protocol will be documented in memo to file.

16.0 Health and Safety Requirements

All the personnel involving in sample processing are vaccinated with Hepatitis B vaccine. While processing samples proper personnel protective equipment like, face mask, head caps, gloves, apron are worn to reduce the risk of potentially infectious materials. Fire extinguisher, emergency shower, eye wash fountains are in the lab and periodic functional checks are documented.

Chapter 7

Summary

In the present book, mainly following things were tried to elaborate:

- Rules and regulations of establishment and functioning of A CRO (Bioequivalence Study Centre) in India.
- Requirements of the detailed methodology along with necessary documents in conducting of a Bioequivalence Study. A case study of montelukast 10 mg has been discussed elaborately in the different chapters.

It's been evident from the previous chapters, what are the requirements of establishment and functioning of a Bioequivalence Study Centre.

Moreover, from the management perspective it should be noted that:

- ❖ **QA/QC:** Quality Control and Quality Assurance needs to be maintained though out the study. The Critical steps of a particular study need to be identified and properly monitored to assure the integrity of the generated data and the credibility of the report generated. A quality assurance (QA) monitoring format is attached herewith.
- ❖ **Corrective Action:** Corrective Action elaborates the detailed method of taking corrective actions for eliminating the causes of identified non-conformities in all functional areas by identifying the root causes to prevent their recurrence and to ensure that the proposed corrective actions are effective (Attached herewith as **Appendix-I**).
- ❖ **Preventive Action:** This procedure details the method of taking preventive actions through analysis of quality records and applying controls to prevent occurrence of potential non-conformities/problems and to ensure that the proposed preventive actions are effective and appropriate to the effects of identified potential problems (Attached herewith as **Appendix-II**).
- ❖ **Training of the Employees:** Proper training should be arranged for the staffs of different departments according to the time specified in the relevant SOP. It should be noted that the BA/BE Study has to be carried out under strict regulatory environment, and regulatory guidelines is changing or updating day to day. So if the top management plans and provides the necessary external and internal

training to the employees, they can withstand to the regulatory requirements. A sample copy of the training programme schedule is furnished below:

Tentative Training Schedule of Employees

Training Calendar

Jan	Feb	Mar	Apr	May	Jun	Jul	Aug	Sept	Oct	Nov	Dec
Analysis/ Analytical Process*											
	Scientific Writing/ Documentation*										
			Changes/Updates in Regulatory Guidelines*								
					Bio-analytical*						
Instrumental Analysis/ Bio-analysis#					GCP Training#				Training by the Sponsor/Industry Experts#		
							Analysis/ Analytical Process*				
								Scientific Writing/ Documentation*			
									Changes/Updates in Regulatory Guidelines*		
										Bio-analytical*	

Internal Training----* and External Training---#

❖ **Archival Management**: There are two basic methods of storing and retrieving records in general. These methods are --**Manual & Electronic**.

➢   **Manual Storage System**

It involves keeping records of various activities performed at different stages in written form in the following formats

I.   Files/ Copy of Reports

II.   Registers

III. Log Book

IV. Different Forms

V.   Investigational Product (IP)

It should be noted that, all entries should be made in a legible and orderly manner using permanent ink. Make entries clear and complete. Avoid erasures. If an error is made, cross it out and make the correction immediately thereafter. Cancellations or insertions should be initialed, dated and explained (in the margin, if possible), by an appropriate notation. State the object and results of each experiment clearly and concisely. Negative or disparaging entries should be avoided. Each day's work should be noted in the particular logbook when the work has been completed in continuation from the last entry of the same notebook. Each entry must be signed and dated by the individual who makes the entry and does the work. Where two or more individuals make a conception, it need only be entered in the notebook of one. Report the loss of theft of a research notebook. Following the use of all the pages of each Laboratory Notebook, it should be sent to the QA Department for record maintenance and another notebook will be issued for that process.

➢ **Electronic Storage System**

Electronic Records are records in electronic form that are created, modified, maintained, archived, retrieved, or transmitted under any requirements set forth in regulatory authority regulations. (FDA Definition)

The devices used for storing the electronic data include:

I. Personal Computers (Desktops, laptops etc)

II. Compact disc (CD) etc.

Format for Drug Accountability Register

Study No:			
Study Drug:			
Sponsor:		**Receive Date:**	
Test Drug Information	**Trade/Brand Name**		
	MFG By:		
	MFG and Exp Date:		
	Batch No.:		
	Quantity Received:		
Reference Drug Information	**Trade/Brand Name**		
	MFG By:		
	MFG and Exp Date:		
	Batch No.:		
	Quantity Received:		
Dissolution Study Details	**Study Date:**		**Signature**
Quantity Dispensed:	Test:	Reference:	
Phase-I (Period-I) Study Details		**Date:**	
			Signature
Samples Dispensed for P-I Study:	Test:	Reference:	
Phase-II (Period-II) Study Details		**Date:**	
			Signature
Samples Dispensed for P-II Study:	Test:	Reference:	
Remaining Samples after P-I & P-II			**Signature**
	Test (T):		
	Reference (R):		

All data and report must be prepared in the MS WORD and MS EXCEL and should be kept in doc format, pdf format and excel spread sheet. In case any other software used the name and version of the software used must be documented properly so that the data can be reproduced, if required. No editing is permissible after submission of the report and regarding documents. Files and folders should be properly entitled and indexed should be maintained. All the computers where data being recorded should be password protected in order to protect pilferage and two/three personnel will be authorised to access the computers.

As per the Indian regulatory requirements BE Study Reports have to be archived for 5 years. The investigational products have to be archived for 3 years or till the expiry date of the drug. But the above regulatory requirements have to be implement according to the agreement between the CRO and Sponsor.

List of Annexures:

- **Appendix-I:** Corrective Action Plan
- **Appendix-II:** Preventive Action Plan

Document Title	**CORRECTIVE ACTION**	Issue No	
		Effective Date	
		Revision Date	
Document Number		Revision Number	

Sl.	Contents	Page No
1	**Purpose**	2
2	**Scope**	2
3	**Related Documents**	2
4	**Responsibility**	2
5	**Data Source**	3
6	**Methodology for Corrective Actions & Corrective Action for Controlling of Process Flow Sheet**	3
7	**Verification on Implementation**	6
8	**Quality Records**	6

Distribution Control Status		Master copy		
Issue & Controlled by	Management Representative	Approved by		Page 1/5
Signature		Signature		
Name		Name		

Document Title	CORRECTIVE ACTION	Issue No	
		Effective Date	
		Revision Date	
Document Number		Revision Number	

1. PURPOSE

This procedure details the method of taking corrective actions for eliminating the causes of identified non-conformities in all functional areas by identifying the root causes to prevent their recurrence and to ensure that the proposed corrective actions are effective.

2. SCOPE

This procedure is applicable when non-conformance are revealed and disposed of as per quality-system procedure, Non-conformance control QSP 83 or as a result of internal quality audits as per quality system procedure Internal Quality Audits QSP S22 Corrective actions arc applicable for the entire organization and product/operation range.

3. RELATED DOCUMENTS
CDSCO Guidelines, New Delhi
Quality System Procedure - Nonconformate control QSP S3
Quality System Procedure - Internal Quality Audit QSPR22

4. RESPONSIBILITY

SI. No	Record	Responsibility
1	NCR-Corrective action - closing of NCR	Auditee/HOD & Team Leader responsible/ Internal auditor/MR
2	List of problems	MR/concerned HOD & Team Leader responsible
3	Problem solving action plan	HOD & Team Leader responsible
4	Request for change - specification/document	Concerned personnel /MR
5	Training request	HOD & Team Leader responsible
6	Customer complaints	

The above generally defines all responubility. However, any or all above may designate or solicit assistance from any other source to ensure satisfactory conclusion.

Distribution Control Status		Master copy		
Issue & Controlled by	Management Representative	Approved by		Page 2/5
Signature		Signature		
Name		Name		

Document Title	CORRECTIVE ACTION	Issue No	
		Effective Date	
		Revision Date	
Document Number		Revision Number	

4.1 All HODs hold primary responsibility to implement corrective actions in respective functional areas covering all activities and concerning all employees of the respective departments. In case, corrective actions are needed in system procedures, the Management Representative is responsible to find alternative better methods and procedures.

4.2 In overlapping situations appropriate personnel are specifically authorized to implement solutions.

5. DATA SOURCE

Following records are data sources to identify non-conformances.

5.1 Internal failures

(i) Test reports

(ii) Non-conformance report Machinery breakdown reports

(iii) Scrap reports

(iv) Audit reports

(v) Statistical analysis reports

5.2 External failures

(i) Customer complaint reports
(ii) Minutes of meeting with customer
(iii) Users view on quality
(iv) Minutes of meeting of Management Review Committee

6. METHODOLOGY OF CORRECTIVE ACTIONS

Corrective actions are implemented after analysis of non-conformance with a view to eliminate the root cause and control reoccurrence.

Distribution Control Status		Master copy		
Issue & Controlled by	Management Representative	Approved by		Page 3/5
Signature		Signature		
Name		Name		

Document Title	CORRECTIVE ACTION	Issue No	
		Effective Date	
		Revision Date	
Document Number		Revision Number	

CORRECTIVE ACTION FOR CONTROLLING
OF PROCESS FLOW SHEET

Reviewing of all detected nonconformities in process, procedure, quality, customer service, QMS jointly by HOBs and MR

↓

Analyzing detected/identified non-conformity/problem both from internal & external source

↓

Determining the causes of identified nonconformities in respective dept. by HODs

↓

Evaluating need for action to ensure non-recurrence and QMS

↓

Determining actions to eliminate causes of non-conformities to prevent recurrence appropriate to the effects of identified non conformities in all functions jointly or individually by HODs & MR

↓

Preparing Action Plan for Implementation of respective Corrective Action by concerned Personnel

↓

Provision of Additional resources by the Top Management, if needed

Distribution Control Status		Master copy		
Issue & Controlled by	Management Representative	Approved by		Page 4/5
Signature		Signature		
Name		Name		

Document Title	CORRECTIVE ACTION	Issue No	
		Effective Date	
		Revision Date	
Document Number		Revision Number	

7. VERIFICATION OF IMPLEMENTATION

7.1 Once a solution to potential problem/noncompliance is identified a target date/time frame is fixed to complete the implementation of proposed preventive action .It is important to identify the organizational interfaces involved and all concerned are to be consulted with regard to the implication of introducing a change.

7.2 The inadequacy of system procedure shall be reported to Management Representative who arranges to amend the same as appropriate.

7.3 In case of preventive actions involving suppliers, the nature of response and manner of implementation of solution by the supplier shall be a major factor for vendor rating. Please refer procedure Departmental Routine Procedure.

7.4 In case of customer suggestions, the systematic handling of customer feedbacks is done by HOD. The above activities are monitored and reviewed periodically.

Delays if any to the programme are intimated to the responsible person for rescheduling. Responsible persons either directly or through their designees ensure that the action as desired has been completed satisfactorily in the stipulated time frame with a note to the MR.

MR maintains status of outstanding preventive actions for reporting in Management Review Meeting.

7.5 Management Review Meeting definitely includes preventive actions (both Proposed and outstanding) prior to being circulated to all areas which may be Effected by the process.

8. RECORDS

- NCRs
- Customer feedback
- List of potential problems and action plans
- Preventive action status
- Management review meeting minutes

Distribution Control Status		Master copy		
Issue & Controlled by	Management Representative	Approved by		
Signature		Signature		Page 5/5
Name		Name		

Document Title	PREVENTIVE ACTION	Issue No	
		Effective Date	
		Revision Date	
Document Number		Revision Number	

Sl.	CONTENTS	Page No
1	**Purpose**	**2**
2	**Scope**	**2**
3	**Related Documents**	**2**
4	**Responsibility**	**2**
5	**Data Source**	**3**
6	**Methodology for Preventive Actions and Preventive Action for Controlling of Process Flow Sheet**	**3**
7	**Verification of Implementation**	**7**
8	**Quality Records**	**8**

Distribution Control Status		Master copy		
Issue & Controlled by	Management Representative	Approved by		Page 1/8
Signature		Signature		
Name		Name		

Document Title	PREVENTIVE ACTION	Issue No	
		Effective Date	
		Revision Date	
Document Number		Revision Number	

1. Purpose

This procedure details the method of taking preventive actions through analysis of quality record's and applying controls to prevent occurrence of potential non-conformities/problems and to ensure that the proposed preventive actions are effective and appropriate to the effects of identified potential problems.

2. Scope

This procedure is applicable when occurrence of potential non-conformance are identified and revealed as a result of prior happenings in similar industries, sector specific experience, technical wisdom, predictions from present operating/production conditions and proposals/opportunities for improvemental (OFI) raised during internal quality audits as per quality system procedure-Internal Quality Audits QSP 822. Preventive actions are applicable for the entire organization and product operation range.

3. Related Documents

- Quality System Procedure - Internal Quality Audit- QSP

4. Responsibility

Sl.	Record	Responsibility
1	OFI-Preventlve Action -Implementation of proposed preventive action	Officer with overall responsibility Auditee/Head/Team Leader responsible Higher authority /MR
2	List of Potential Problems	All functional Head/Team Leader
3	Problem Solving Action Plan	Concerned Head/Team Leader
4	Request for Change Specification/Document/Procedure	Concerned Personnel/MR/Concerned Head/Team Leader
5	Training Request	Concerned Head/Team Leader

Distribution Control Status		**Master copy**		
Issue & Controlled by	Management Representative	**Approved by**		Page 2/8
Signature		**Signature**		
Name		**Name**		

Document Title	PREVENTIVE ACTION	Issue No	
		Effective Date	
		Revision Date	
Document Number		Revision Number	

4.1 The MR in liaison with top management higher authority and respective HOB holds primary responsibility to propose/ finalize / implement preventive actions in case of all activities and concerning all employees of all departments and company as a whole, In case, preventive actions are needed in system procedures ,the management representative. HOB is responsible to find alternative better methods and procedures appropriate to the particular activity/function.

4.3 In overlapping situations appropriate personnel are specifically authorized to implement preventive solutions.

5. Data Source

Following records are data sources to identify non-conformances.

5.1 Internal source
I. Non-conformance report indicating OFI's.
II. Routine preventive maintenance report of machinery/equipment.
III. Reports on near misses in the factory.
IV. Audit reports.
V. Technical wisdom of experts.
VI. Knowledge and prior experience of company personnel in similar industry.
VII. Statistical analysis reports.

5.2 External source
I. Customer feedback reports (indicating preventive suggestions).
II. Service engineers report on prevention.
III. Minutes of meeting with customer.
IV. Users view on quality.
V. Minutes of meeting of management review committee,
VI. Report on mishaps in similar industries.

Distribution Control Status		Master copy			
Issue & Controlled by	Management Representative	Approved by			Page
Signature		Signature			3/8
Name		Name			

Document Title	PREVENTIVE ACTION	Issue No	
		Effective Date	
		Revision Date	
Document Number		Revision Number	

Preventive actions are implemented after analysis of reports from the above source with a view to eliminate the probability/possibility of occurrence.

6. Methodology of Preventive Actions

Preventive action is only initiated to improve a given system already existing in the organization or when certain eventualities like near miss events are reported to eliminate potential non-conformity.

PREVENTIVE ACTION FOR CONTROLLING OF PROCESS FLOW SHEET

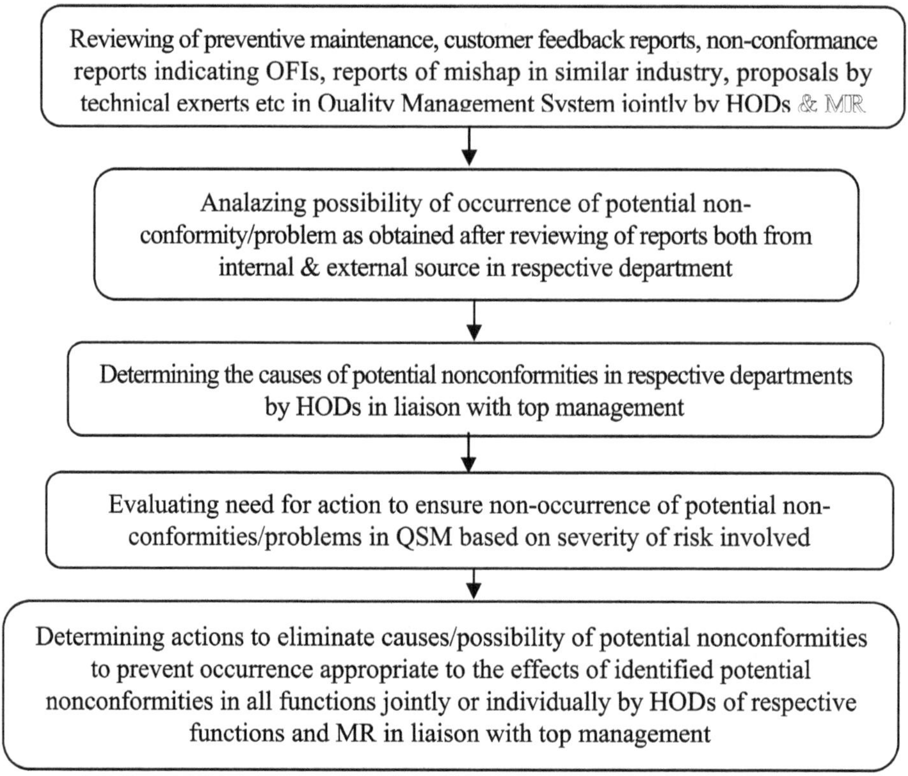

Reviewing of preventive maintenance, customer feedback reports, non-conformance reports indicating OFIs, reports of mishap in similar industry, proposals by technical experts etc in Quality Management System jointly by HODs & MR

↓

Analazing possibility of occurrence of potential non-conformity/problem as obtained after reviewing of reports both from internal & external source in respective department

↓

Determining the causes of potential nonconformities in respective departments by HODs in liaison with top management

↓

Evaluating need for action to ensure non-occurrence of potential non-conformities/problems in QSM based on severity of risk involved

↓

Determining actions to eliminate causes/possibility of potential nonconformities to prevent occurrence appropriate to the effects of identified potential nonconformities in all functions jointly or individually by HODs of respective functions and MR in liaison with top management

Distribution Control Status		Master copy		
Issue & Controlled by	Management Representative	Approved by		Page
Signature		Signature		4/8
Name		Name		

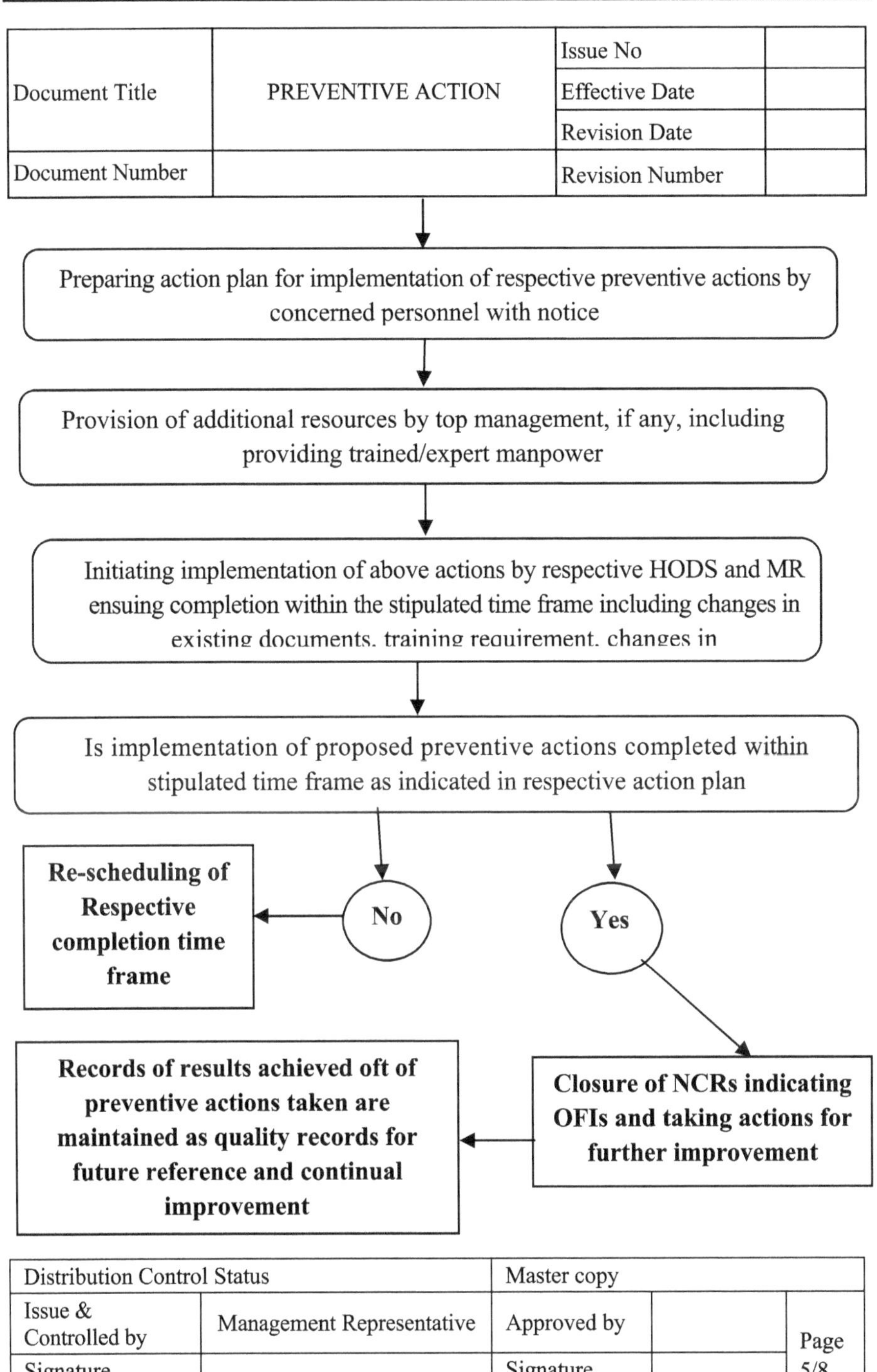
Document Title
PREVENTIVE ACTION
Issue No
Effective Date
Revision Date
Document Number
Revision Number
Preparing action plan for implementation of respective preventive actions by concerned personnel with notice
Provision of additional resources by top management, if any, including providing trained/expert manpower
Initiating implementation of above actions by respective HODS and MR ensuing completion within the stipulated time frame including changes in existing documents, training requirement, changes in
Is implementation of proposed preventive actions completed within stipulated time frame as indicated in respective action plan
Re-scheduling of Respective completion time frame
No
Yes
Records of results achieved oft of preventive actions taken are maintained as quality records for future reference and continual improvement
Closure of NCRs indicating OFIs and taking actions for further improvement
Distribution Control Status
Master copy
Issue & Controlled by
Management Representative
Approved by
Signature
Signature
Name
Name
Page 5/8

Document Title	PREVENTIVE ACTION	Issue No	
		Effective Date	
		Revision Date	
Document Number		Revision Number	

6.1 The methodology adopted varies depending on the nature of potential problem and the relative easiness with which the causes can be identified, the risk involved, the status and importance of the potential non-conformity, etc.

6.2 MR and all HOD's analyses the data sources at least once in six months through suitable statistical techniques to identify potential problems and their causes based on the increase in the possibility of number of incidents till failures otherwise and the list of potential problems is discussed in MRC meeting.

6.3 The root causes which are generally hidden are understood based on experience gained in problem solving and a course of action is planned and officer having overall responsibility initiates the same, which may include:

(a) Training request

(b) Request for change in specification

(c) Request for change in document

(d) Full proofing of the process/change on the process plan

(e) Introduction of statistical technique

6.4 List of problem and action plan

All the HOD's periodically submit to MR a list of potential problems. If any identified with respective action plan after analysing available reports based on discussions with concerned officers along with a time frame for preventive actions indicating priorities (long term/short term).Potential problems, plans and actions are reviewed at least once in six months in Management Review Committee Meeting.

- Customer's constructive suggestion reports arising out of analysis of customer's feedback is copied to the responsible personnel detailed above for proposing suitable and practical preventive actions,

- Analysis of the reports from above sources are carried out and the action arising out of these discussions are noted,

Distribution Control Status		Master copy		
Issue & Controlled by	Management Representative	Approved by		Page 6/8
Signature		Signature		
Name		Name		

Document Title	PREVENTIVE ACTION	Issue No	
		Effective Date	
		Revision Date	
Document Number		Revision Number	

- The sequencing and selection of potential problems for immediate initiation of preventive action is done judiciously commensurate with the potential risk encountered.

Preventive action could result in any one or more of the following actions:

- Amendments to documented procedures
- Amendments in routine/regular practices
- Changes to preventive maintenance schedule
- Adoption of better advanced techniques
- Additional orientation and training and others

6.5   Action plan for problem solving

Preventive actions required are intimated to the person concerned through respective Heads/Team Leaders who would be required to implement the same in lime hound manner. Top management ensures the availability of additional resources including trained manpower or effective implementation of proposed preventive actions. Alt preventive actions are ensured to be implemented within the accepted time frame; however the duration of implementation would be at the discretion of the respective Heads/Team Leaders depending upon the severity of the potential non-compliance/problems.

6.6 In ease the potential problem needs detailed analysis, a problem solving action plan for concerned problem is generated, as appropriate. After discussion with concerned employees who can contribute to identify the potential causes. A sequence of solutions arc selected based on an agreed action plan. The action plan is forwarded to all concerned and the plan updated till the problem concerned is effectively sorted out.

6.7 Through NCR Forms: The originator (auditor) of NCR takes up with the auditee and mutually agrees on the proposed opportunity for improvements (OFIs) and accordingly the NCR form is filled up with a proposed time frame for implementation in liaison with MR/Top management, The originator verifies the status and confirms that preventive action is implemented or appropriate actions against proposed OFIs adopted/practiced.

Distribution Control Status		Master copy		
Issue & Controlled by	Management Representative	Approved by		Page 7/8
Signature		Signature		
Name		Name		

		Issue No	
Document Title	PREVENTIVE ACTION	Effective Date	
		Revision Date	
Document Number		Revision Number	

7. Verification of Implementation:

7.1 Once a solution to potential problem/noncompliance is identified a target date/time frame is fixed to complete the implementation of proposed preventive action. It is important to identify the organizational interfaces involved and all concerned are to be consulted with regard to the implication of introducing a change.

7.2 The inadequacy of system procedure shall be reported to Management Representative who arranges to amend the same as appropriate.

7.3 In case of preventive actions involving suppliers the nature of response and manner of implementation of solution by the supplier shall be a major factor for vendor rating.

7.4 In case of customer suggestions, the systematic handling of customer feedbacks is done by Heads/Team Leaders. The above activities are monitored and reviewed periodically. Delays if any to the programme are intimated to the responsible person for rescheduling. Responsible persons either directly or through their designees ensure that the action as desired has been completed satisfactorily in the stipulated lime frame with a note to the MR. MR maintains status of outstanding preventive actions for reporting in Management Review Meeting.

7.5 Management Review Meeting definitely includes preventive actions (both Proposed and outstanding) prior to being circulated to all areas which may be Effected by the process.

Distribution Control Status		Master copy		
Issue & Controlled by	Management Representative	Approved by		Page 8/8
Signature		Signature		
Name		**Name**		

Chapter 8

LC-MS/MS Instrumentation

Liquid Chromatography Mass Spectrometry (LC-MS/MS) Instrumentation

Introduction

Liquid chromatography–mass spectrometry (LC-MS) is an analytical chemistry technique that combines the physical separation capabilities of liquid chromatography (or HPLC) with the mass analysis capabilities of mass spectrometry (MS).

In general, liquid chromatography (LC) separates the components of a sample based on differences in their affinity (or retention strength) for the stationary phase or mobile phase, then detects the separated components using UV, fluorescence, or electrical conductivity based on their properties. Such detectors primarily qualify substances based on retention time and quantitate substances based on peak intensity and peak area. Chromatography offers great resolution, but accurately qualifying and quantitating substances can be difficult if multiple components elute approximately at the same time, such as during simultaneous multianalyte analysis. Whereas, mass spectrometry (MS) offers a highly sensitive detection technique that ionizes the sample components using various methods, then separates the resulting ions in vacuum based on their mass-to-charge ratios and measures the intensity of each ion. Since the mass spectra provided by MS can indicate the concentration level of ions that have a given mass, it is extremely helpful for qualitative analysis. That is because mass is information particular to specific molecules and MS enables obtaining that information directly.

With LC-MS, solubilized compounds (the mobile phase) are passed through a column packed with a stationary (solid) phase. This effectively separates the compounds based on their molecular weight and affinity for the mobile and stationary phases of the column.

A flow diagram of LC-MS/MS along with its accessories is schematically represented in the following figure-1.

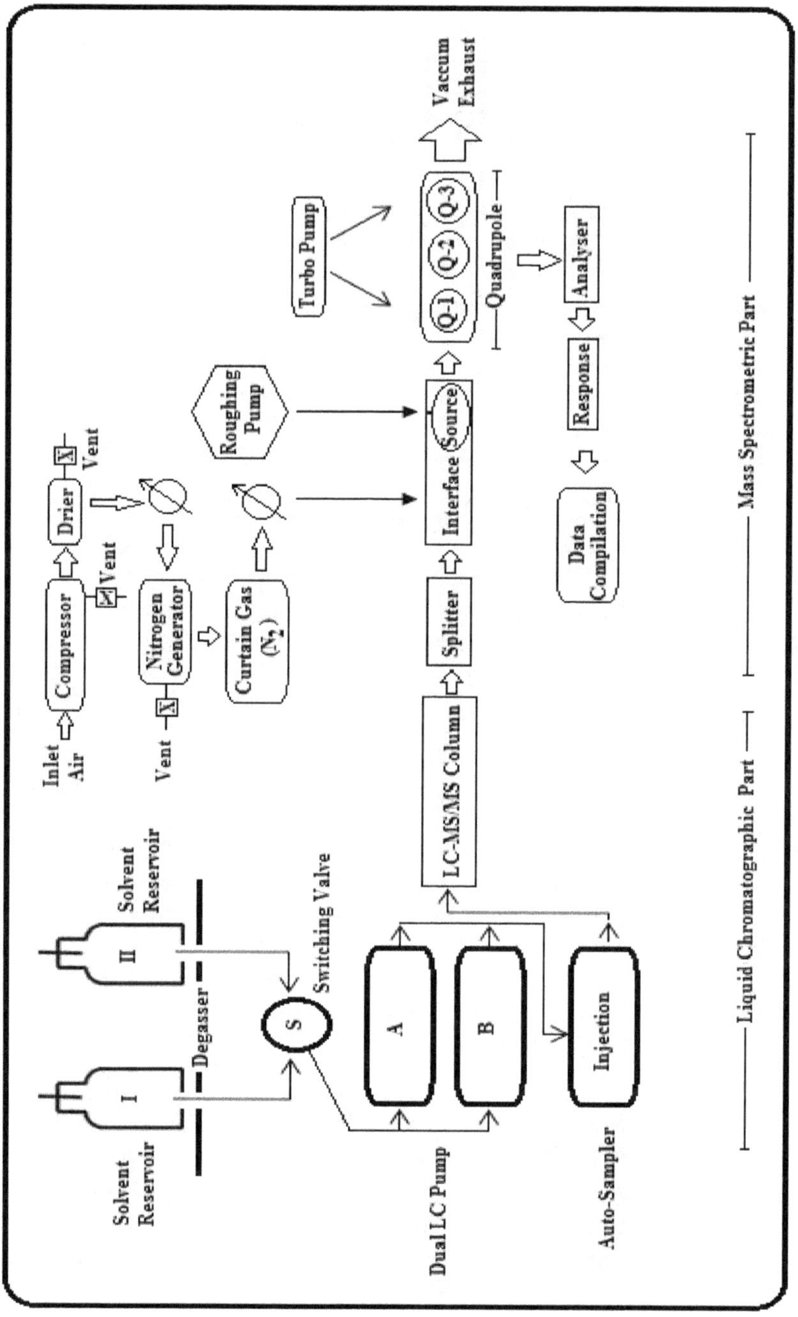

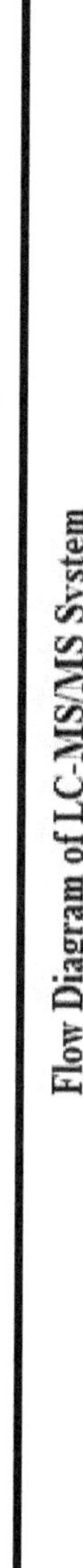

Figure 1 Flow Diagram of LC-MS/MS System

Key Process Involved in a LC-MS/MS System

- **Ion Production:** Atmospheric pressure ionization (API)
- **Transition to Vacuum:** Ions pass through the Curtain Gas interface between atmospheric pressure and vacuum.
- **m/z-Selection in a quadruple (Q), Linear Ion Trap (LIT), and Time-of-Flight (TOF) mass analyzer:**
  - ✓ Ion selection according to their m/z values (Q1, Q3)
  - ✓ Ion trapping and scanning in a LIT
  - ✓ Ion selection in a TOF
- **MS/MS fragmentation in a collision cell (Q2)**
- **Detection:** Ion detection using an electron multiplier
- **Signal and data processing**

Different Types of Ion Production Process

A. **Electrospray Ionization (ESI):** Ionization by high voltage in liquid phase (droplet)

B. **Atmospheric Pressure Chemical Ionization (APCI):** Chemical Ionization in gas phase

C. **Atmospheric Pressure Photo Ionization (APPI):** Ionization by UV light

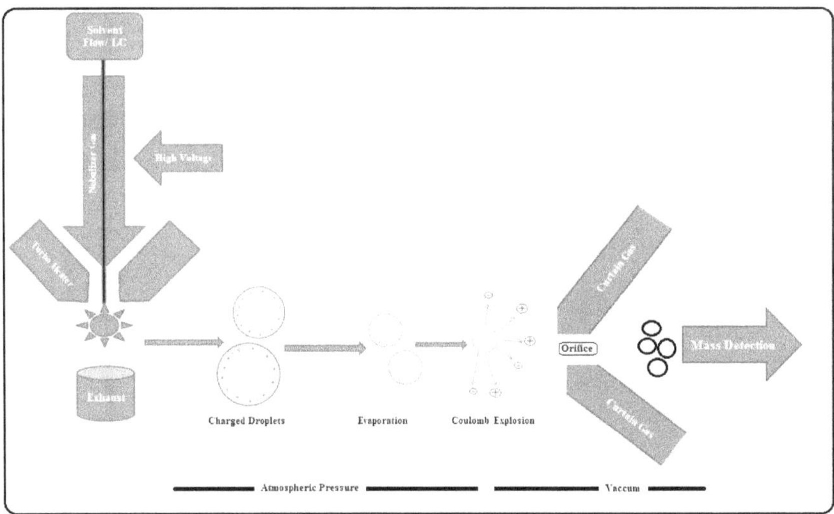

Schematic Diagram of Trubo Source (ESI)

Figure 2 Turbo Source (ESI)

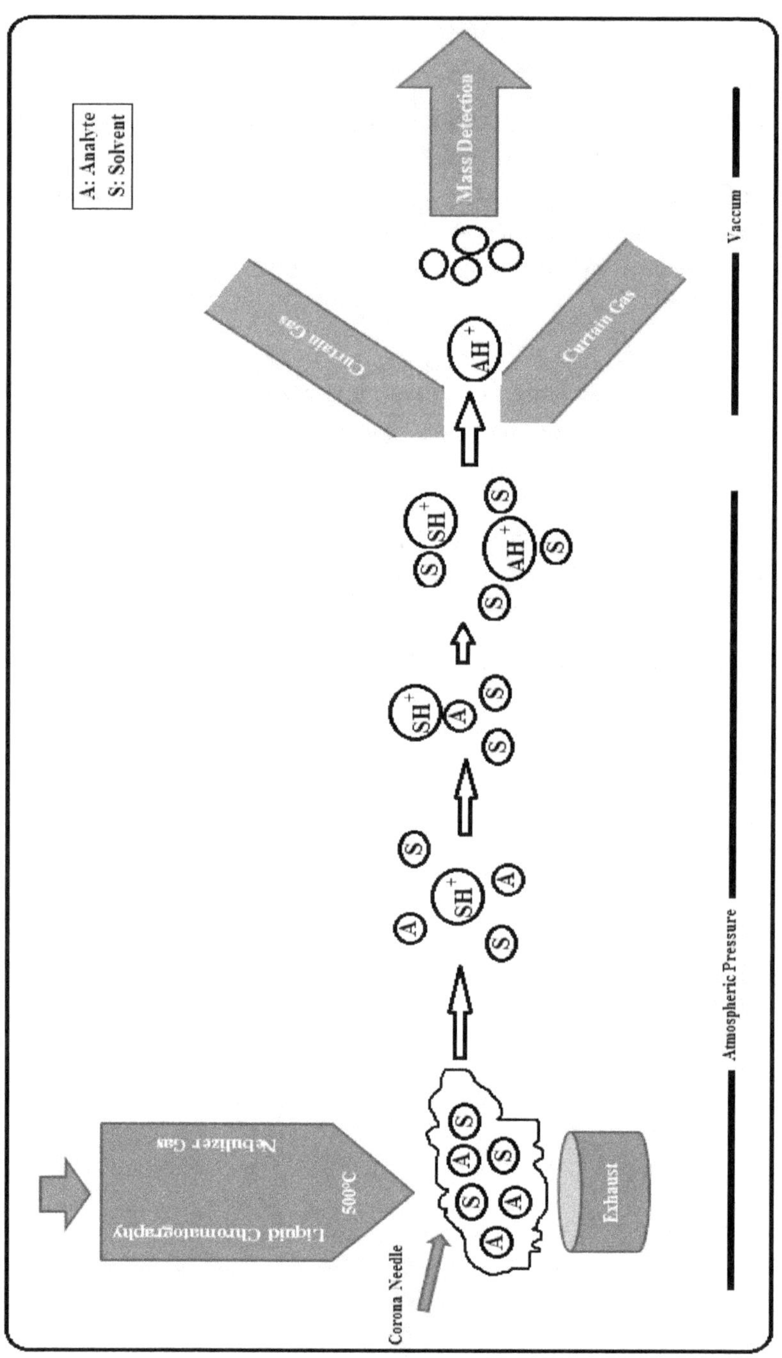

Figure 3 Turbo Source (APCI)

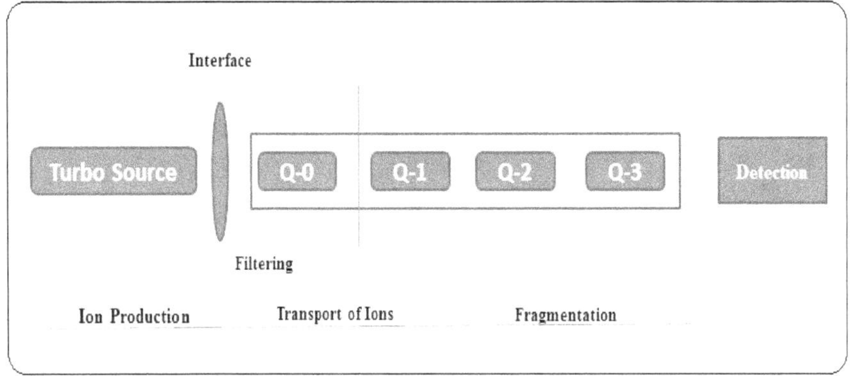

Figure 4 General Setup of a Triple Quadruple Instrument

Operating Parameters of LC-MS/MS Accessories

Accessories	Description	Specifications
Compressor	Single stage low pressure compressor	2-3 HP; 6-8 kg/cm^2
Drier	Removes moisture, other organic vapor and particles (0.1-3 micron) by two filters (GP and ZP)	2-4 °C
Nitrogen Generator	Compressed air enters from the drier as source which separates as two components (O_2 and N_2) through membrane filter as curtain gas and exhaust	Operating Pressure of A) Curtain Gas: 50 psi B) Exhaust: 45 psi C) Source: 100 psi

Various Accessories of LCMS/MS

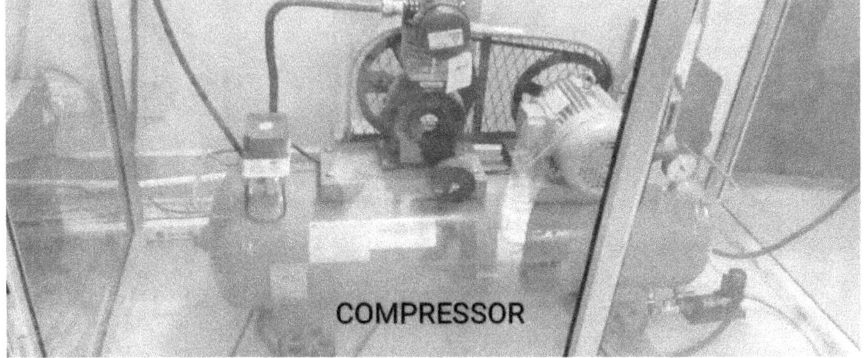

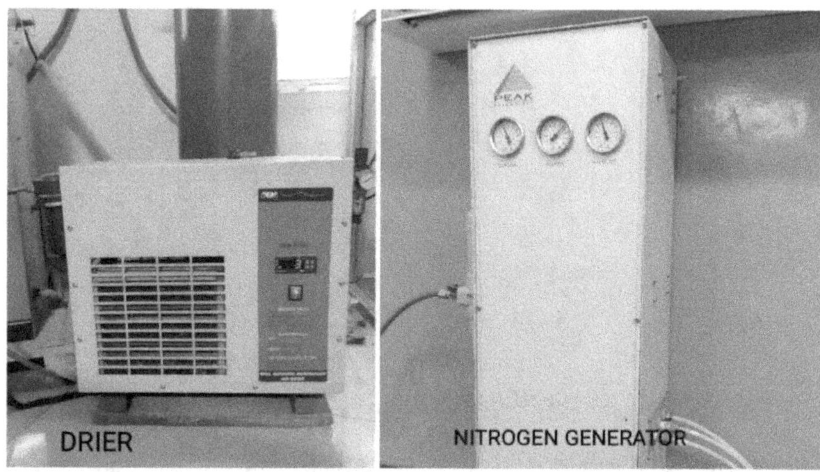
DRIER
NITROGEN GENERATOR

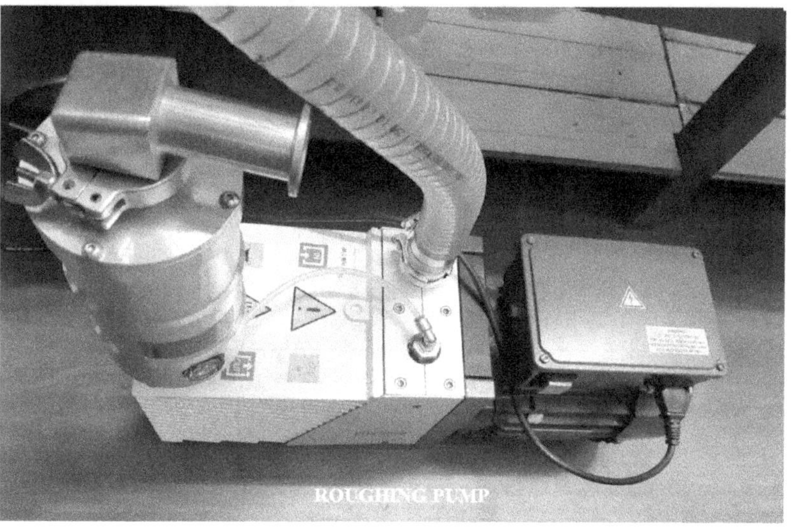
ROUGHING PUMP

Chapter 9
References & Appendices

The following guidelines, articles, notices and office orders may be consulted for further information.

* Central Drugs Standard Control Organization (CDSCO), Drugs and Cosmetics Rules. 1945. Available from: http://cdsco.nic.in/html/D&C_Rules_Schedule_Y.pdf.

* Central Drugs Standard Control Organization (CDSCO, Govt. of India). Guidelines for BA/BE Study. http://cdsco.nic.in/forms/list.aspx?lid=1855andId=1.

* Amendment to the Drugs & Cosmetics Rules-1945, Gazette Notification [GSR 72 (E)] dated 8th February 2013. http://cdsco.nic.in/html/G.S.R%2072 (E) % 20 dated % 2008.02.2013.pdf.

* Central Drugs Standard Control Organization (CDSCO): Good Clinical Practices for Clinical Research in India.2013.

* Central Drugs Standard Control Organization (CDSCO), Notice of proposal for creation of IT enabled system.

* Central Drugs Standard Control Organization (CDSCO), Guidance for Audio Visual Recording. (2014).

* Actions on the recommendations of Prof. Ranjit Roy Chaudhury expert committee to formulate policy and guidelines for approval of new drugs, clinical trials and banning of drugs. (2013). Accessed from cdsco.nic.in. Action_RR_ Choudhury_Committee.

* Accreditation Standards for Ethics Committee, Investigator, Clinical Trial Site: National Accreditation Board for Hospitals and Healthcare Providers (NABH).

* Guideline for Good Clinical practice. International Conference on Harmonization of Technical Requirements for Registration of pharmaceuticals for Human use. E6 (R1) (1996).

* U. S. Food and Drug Administration. Guidance for Industry: Bioavailability and Bioequivalence Studies for orally Administered Drug Products- General Considerations. Rockville, MD: Center for

Drug Evaluation and Research. 2000. www.fda.gov/downloads/Drugs/.../Guidances/ ucm070124.pdf.

❖ Guidance for Industry Bioanalytical Method Validation. Food and Drug Administration. Center for Drug Evaluation and Research (CDER). United States. 2013.

❖ EMEA. Note for guidance on the investigation of bioavailability and bioequivalence CPMP/EWP/QWP/1401/98; 2002.

❖ European Medicines Agency (EMA). Guidance on Bioanalytical Method Validation, (2012).

❖ Ethical guidelines for biomedical research on human participants. New Delhi: Indian Council of Medical Research, 2006. http://icmr.nic.in/ethical_ guidelines.pdf.

❖ World Medical Association. The Declaration of Helsinki. http://www.wma.net/en/ 30publications/10policies/b3.

❖ Ethics Committee Registration Letter of CDSCO, New Delhi, India. Available from: http://cdsco.nic.in/ECR%20103.pdf.

❖ Dan S., Ghosh B., Gorain B. and Pal T. K. Mandatory Registration of the Research Ethics Committees in India. *Applied Clinical Research, Clinical Trials and Regulatory Affairs.* 2014. 1. 88-92.

❖ Dan S, Karmakar S, Ghosh B, Pal TK. (2015). Digitization of Clinical Trials in India: A New Step by CDSCO towards Ensuring the Data Credibility and Patient Safety. Pharmaceut Reg Affairs. 4: 149. doi:10.4172/21677689.1000149.

❖ Shubhasis Dan, Hira Choudhury, Bapi Gorain, Pradipto Sarkar, Anwesha Barik, Balaram Ghosh and Tapan Kumar Pal. A randomized two-way crossover comparative Pharmacokinetics study of two different tablet formulations containing Ilaprazole in healthy human Indian volunteers. Archives of Medicine and Health Sciences. 2014; 2:160-4. [www.amhsjournal.org].

❖ Shubhasis Dan, Dhiman Halder, Anwesha Barik, Easha Biswas, Murari Mohun Pal, Balaram Ghosh, Pradipta Sarkar, Chinmoy Das, Pragnya Chakraborty, Sangujkta Pradhan and Tapan Kumar Pal. Bio-analytical Method Development and Validation of Tadalafil with a Special Emphasis on pharmacokinetic Study in Healthy Indian Subjects for the ODS Formulation. Current Analytical Chemistry. 2015, 11, 175-183. [DOI: 10.2174/1573411011666150219203105].

❖ Shubhasis Dan, Dhiman Halder, Anwesha Barik, Easha Biswas, Pragnya Chakraborty, Pradipta Sarkar, Murari Mohan Pal, Chinmoy Das, Rubina Bose, Balaram Ghosh and Tapan Kumar

Pal. Comparative Bioavailability Study of Two Antiretroviral FDC Containing Abacavir 600 mg and Lamivudine 300 mg in Healthy Human Indian Volunteers. Journal of Applied Biopharmaceutics and Pharmacokinetics, 2015, 3, 18-26. DOI: http://dx.doi.org/10.14205/2309-4435.2015.03.01.3.

❖ Dhiman Halder, Shubhasis Dan, Easha Biswas, Pradipta Sarkar, Umesh C. Halder and Tapan K. Pal. A Rapid LC-ESI-MS/MS Method for the Quantitation of Salicylic Acid, an Active Metabolite of Acetylsalicylic Acid: Application to in vivo Pharmacokinetic and Bioequivalence Study in Indian Healthy Male Volunteers. Applied Clinical Research, Clinical Trials & Regulatory Affairs, 2015, 2 (2). 90–102. [DOI: 10.2174/2213476X03666151105185505].

❖ Dhiman Halder, Shubhasis Dan, Murari Mohan Pal, Easha Biswas, Nilendra Chatterjee, Pradipta Sarkar, Umesh Chandra Halder and Tapan Kumar Pal. LC–MS/MS assay for quantitation of enalapril and enalaprilat in plasma for bioequivalence study in Indian subjects. Future Sci. OA. (2017), 3 (1). [DOI: 10.4155/fsoa-2016-0071].

❖ Hira Choudhury, Bapi Gorain, Anwesha Paul, Pradipta Sarkar, Shubhasis Dan, Pragnya Chakraborty, Tapan Kumar Pal. Development and validation of an LC-MS/MS-ESI method for comparative pharmacokinetic study of ciprofloxacin in healthy male subjects. *Arzneimittel forschung/ Drug Research.* (2016); 66: 1–8. [DOI http://dx.doi.org/10.1055/s-0042-116593].

❖ Mandal Pallab, Dan Shubhasis, Ghosh Balaram, Barma Sujata, Bose Rubina and Pal Tapan Kumar. Simultaneous Determination and Quantitation of Metformin and Teneligliptin in human plasma by LC-ESI-MS/MS with an application to pharmacokinetic studies. *Indian Drugs.* 55 (04) 27-38. April 2018.

GUIDELINES FOR BIOAVAILABILITY & BIOEQUIVALENCE STUDIES

Central Drugs Standard Control Organization,

Directorate General of Health Services,

Ministry of Health & Family Welfare,

Government of India,

New Delhi.

(March 2005)

These guidelines should be read in conjunction with Schedule Y to the Drugs and Cosmetic Rules, GCP Guidelines issued by CDSCO, Ministry of Health and Family Welfare, GLP and the Ethical Guidelines for Biomedical research on human subjects issued by Indian Council of Medical Research. All provisions described in above documents shall appropriately apply to the conduct of bioavailability and bioequivalence studies.

Contents

1. INTRODUCTION

2. DEFINITIONS

3. SCOPE OF THE GUIDELINES

   3.1   When bioequivalence studies are necessary and types of studies required

   3.1.1. In vivo studies

   3.1.2. In vitro studies

   3.2   When bioequivalence studies are not necessary

4. DESIGN AND CONDUCT OF STUDIES

   4.1   Pharmacokinetic Studies

   4.1.1. Study design

   4.1.2. Study population

   4.1.3. Study conditions

   4.1.4. Characteristics to be investigated

   4.1.5. Bioanalytical methodology

   4.1.6. Statistical evaluation

   4.1.7. Special considerations for modified release drug products

   i   Study parameters

   ii   Study design

   iii   Requirements for modified release drug products unlikely to accumulate

   iv   Requirements for modified release drug products likely to accumulate

   4.2   Pharmacodynamic Studies

   4.3. Comparative Clinical Trials

   4.4. In-vitro Studies

5. DOCUMENTATION

6. FACILITIES FOR CONDUCTING BA/BE STUDIES

7. MAINTENANCE OF RECORDS OF BA/BE STUDIES

8. RETENTION OF BA/BE SAMPLES

9. SPECIAL TOPICS

    9.1. Food effect bioavailability studies

    9.2. Long half life drugs

    9.3. Early Exposure

    9.4. Individual and population bioequivalence

1. INTRODUCTION

Ensuring uniformity in standards of quality, efficacy and safety of pharmaceutical products is the fundamental responsibility of CDSCO. Reasonable assurance has to be provided that various products, containing same active ingredients, marketed by different licensees, are clinically equivalent and interchangeable.

Accordingly, the bioavailability of an active substance from a pharmaceutical product should be known and reproducible. In most cases, it is cumbersome and unnecessary to assess this by clinical studies. Bioavailability and bioequivalence data is therefore required to be furnished with applications for new drugs, as required under Schedule Y, depending on the type of application being submitted.

Both bioavailability and bioequivalence focus on the release of a drug substance from its dosage form and subsequent absorption into the systemic circulation. For this reason, similar approaches to measuring bioavailability should generally be followed in demonstrating bioequivalence.

Bioavailability can be generally documented by a systemic exposure profile obtained by measuring drug and/or metabolite concentration in the systemic circulation over time. The systemic exposure profile determined during clinical trials in the early drug development can serve as a benchmark for subsequent BE studies.

Bioequivalence studies should be conducted for the comparison of two medicinal products containing the same active substance. The studies should provide an objective means of critically assessing the possibility of alternative use of them. Two products marketed by different licensees, containing same active ingredient(s), must be shown to be therapeutically equivalent to one another in order to be considered interchangeable. Several test methods are available to assess equivalence, including:

i   comparative bioavailability (bioequivalence) studies, in which the active drug substance or one or more metabolites is measured in an accessible biological fluid such as plasma, blood or urine

ii   comparative pharmacodynamic studies in humans

iii   comparative clinical trials

iv   in-vitro dissolution tests

The guidelines describe when bioavailability or bioequivalence studies are necessary and describe requirements for their design, conduct, and evaluation.

The possibility of using *in vitro* instead of *in vivo* studies with pharmacokinetic end points is also envisaged.

For classes of products, including many biologicals such as vaccines, animal sera, and products derived from human blood and plasma, and product manufactured by biotechnology, the concept of interchangeability raises complex which may be addressed by the applicant on the basis of contemporary scientific rationale.

In vivo bioequivalence/bioavailability studies recommended for approval of modified release products should be designed to ensure that

I   the product meets the modified release label claims

ii   the product does not release the active drug substance at a rate and extent leading to dose dumping

iii there is no significant difference between the performance of the modified release product and the reference product, when given in dosage regimes to arrive at the steady state.

Iv   there must be a significant difference between the performance of modified release product and the conventional release product when used as reference product.

It is appreciated that pharmacokinetic studies can be conducted during any phase of a clinical trial for New Chemical Entities (NCEs). While these guidelines deal with pharmacokinetic/ pharmacodynamic studies vis-à-vis bioavailability or bioequivalence studies for a generic drug, the principles described herein, are applicable for any pharmacokinetic/ pharmacodynamic study.

2. DEFINITIONS

BIOAVAILABILITY

Bioavailability refers to the relative amount of drug from an administered dosage form which enters the systemic circulation and the rate at which the drug appears in the systemic circulation.

BIOEQUIVALENCE

Bioequivalence of a drug product is achieved if its extent and rate of absorption are not statistically significantly different from those of the reference product when administered at the same molar dose.

CLINICAL TRIAL

A clinical trial is a systematic study of pharmaceutical products in human subject(s), in order to discover or verify the clinical, pharmacological (*including pharmacodynamic / pharmacokinetic*), and/or adverse effects, with the object of determining their safety and/or efficacy.

GOOD CLINICAL PRACTICE (GCP) GUIDELINES:

Good Clinical Practice Guidelines issued by Directorate General of Health Services, Ministry of Health & Family Welfare, Government of India.

MODIFIED RELEASE DOSAGE FORMS

Modified-release dosage forms are those for which the drug-release characteristics of time course and/or drug-release location are chosen to accomplish such therapeutic or convenience objectives that are not offered by immediate-(conventional) release dosage forms.

PHARMACEUTICAL EQUIVALENTS

Pharmaceutical equivalents are drug products that contain identical amounts of the identical active drug ingredient, i.e., the same salt or ester of the same therapeutic moiety, in identical dosage forms, but not necessarily containing the same inactive ingredients.

PHARMACEUTICAL ALTERNATIVES

Pharmaceutical alternatives are drug products that contain the identical therapeutic moiety, or its precursor, but not necessarily in the same amount or dosage form or as the same salt or ester.

PHARMACODYNAMIC EVALUATION

Pharmacodynamic evaluation is measurement of the effect on a pathophysiological process as a function of time, after administration of two different products to serve as a basis for bioequivalence assessment.

PHARMACOKINETICS

Pharmacokinetics deals with the changes of drug concentration in the drug product and changes of concentration of a drug and/or its metabolite(s) in the human or animal body following administration of the drug product, i.e., the changes of drug concentration in the different body fluids and tissues in the dynamic system of liberation, absorption, distribution, body storage, binding, metabolism, and excretion.

NON-LINEAR PHARMACOKINETICS

Nonlinear kinetics or saturation kinetics refers to a change of one or more of the pharmacokinetic parameters during absorption, distribution, metabolism, and excretion by saturation or overloading of processes due to increased dose sizes.

REFERENCE PRODUCT

For purpose of these guidelines, the reference product is a pharmaceutical product which is identified by the Licensing Authority as "Designated Reference Product" and contains the same active ingredient(s) as the new drug. The Designated Reference Product will normally be the global innovator's product. An applicant seeking approval to market a generic equivalent must refer to the Designated Reference Product to which all generic versions must be shown to be bioequivalent. For subsequent new drug applications in India the Licensing Authority may, however, approve another Indian product as Designated Reference Product.

SUPRA-BIOAVAILABILITY

This is a term used when a test product displays an appreciably larger bioavailability than the reference product.

SUSTAINED RELEASE DOSAGE FORM

These are modified release dosage forms where the liberation (drug release) rate constant is smaller than the unrestricted absorption rate constant.

STEADY STATE

Steady state is the state when the plasma concentration of drug at any time point during any dosing interval should be identical to the concentration at the same time during any other dosing interval. The steady state drug concentrations fluctuate (oscillate) between a maximum and a minimum steady state concentration within each of the dosing intervals.

THERAPEUTIC EQUIVALENTS

Therapeutic equivalents are drug products that contain the same active substance or therapeutic moiety and, clinically show the same efficacy and safety.

PHARMACOKINETIC TERMS

C_{max}: This is the maximum drug concentration achieved in systemic circulation following drug administration.

C_{min}: This is the minimum drug concentration achieved in systemic circulation following multiple dosing at steady state.

C_{pd}: This is the pre-dose concentrations determined immediately before a dose is given at steady state.

T_{max}: It is the time required to achieve maximum drug concentration in systemic circulation.

AUC_{0-t}: Area under the plasma concentration - time curve from 0 h to the last quantifiable concentration to be calculated using the trapezoidal rule

$AUC_{0-\infty}$: Area under the plasma concentration - time curve, from zero to infinity to be calculated as the sum of AUC_{0-t} plus the ratio of the last measurable concentration to the elimination rate constant.

$AUC_{0-\tau}$: Area under the plasma concentration - time curve over one dosing interval following single dose for modified release products.

$AUC_{0\tau(ss)}$: Area under the plasma concentration - time curve over one dosing interval in multiple dose study at steady state.

K_{el}: Apparent first-order terminal elimination rate constant calculated from a semi-log plot of the plasma concentration versus time curve.

$T_{1/2}$: Elimination half life of a drug is the time necessary to reduce the drug concentration in the blood, plasma, or serum to one-half after equilibrium is reached.

3. SCOPE OF THE GUIDELINES

Bioavailability and Bioequivalence studies are required by regulations to ensure therapeutic equivalence between a pharmaceutically equivalent test product and a reference product. Several in vivo and in vitro methods are used to measure product quality.

3.1 When bioequivalence studies are necessary and types of studies required

3.1.1 *In vivo* studies

For certain drugs and dosage forms, *in vivo* documentation of equivalence, through either a bioequivalence study, a comparative clinical pharmacodynamic study, or a comparative clinical trial, is regarded as especially important. These include:

a. Oral immediate release drug formulations with systemic action when one or more of the following criteria apply:

   i indicated for serious conditions requiring assured therapeutic response;

   ii narrow therapeutic window/safety margin; steep dose-response curve;

   iii pharmacokinetics complicated by variable or incomplete absorption or absorption window, nonlinear pharmacokinetics, pre-systemic elimination/high first-pass metabolism >70%;

   iv unfavourable physicochemical properties, e.g., low solubility, instability, meta-stable modifications, poor permeability, etc.;

   v documented evidence for bioavailability problems related to the drug or drugs of similar chemical structure or formulations;

   vi where a high ratio of excipients to active ingredients exists.

b. Non-oral and non-parenteral drug formulations designed to act by systemic absorption (such as transdermal patches, suppositories, etc.).

c. Sustained or otherwise modified release drug formulations designed to act by systemic absorption.

d. Fixed-dose combination products with systemic action.

e. Non-solution pharmaceutical products which are for non-systemic use (oral, nasal, ocular, dermal, rectal, vaginal, etc. application) and are intended to act without systemic absorption. In these cases, the bioequivalence concept is not suitable and comparative clinical or pharmacodynamic studies are required to prove equivalence. There is a need for drug concentration measurements in order to assess unintended partial absorption.

Bioequivalence documentation is also needed to establish links between:

    i   early and late clinical trial formulations
    ii formulations used in clinical trials and stability studies, if different
    iii clinical trial formulations and to be marketed drug products
    iv other comparisons, as appropriate

In each comparison, the new formulation or new method of manufacture shall be the test product and the prior formulation (or respective method of manufacture) shall be the reference product.

3.1.2 *In vitro* studies

In following circumstances equivalence may be assessed by the use of *in vitro* dissolution testing:

a. Drugs for which the applicant provides data to substantiate all of the following:

    i. highest dose strength is soluble in 250 ml of an aqueous media over the pH range of 1-7.5 at 37°C

    ii. at least 90% of the administered oral dose is absorbed on mass balance determination or in comparison to an intravenous reference dose

    iii. speed of dissolution as demonstrated by more than 80% dissolution within 15 minutes at 37°C using IP apparatus 1, at 50 rpm or IP apparatus 2, at 100 rpm in a volume of 900 ml or less in each of the following media:

       1. 0.1 N hydrochloric acid or artificial gastric juice (without enzymes)

       2. a pH 4.5 buffer

       3. a pH 6.8 buffer or artificial intestinal juice (without enzymes)

b. Different strengths of the drug manufactured by the same manufacturer, where all of the following criteria are fulfilled:

    i. the qualitative composition between the strengths is essentially the same;

    ii. the ratio of active ingredients and excipients between the strengths is essentially the same, or, in the case of small strengths, the ratio between the excipients is the same;

    iii. the method of manufacture is essentially the same;

    iv. an appropriate equivalence study has been performed on at least one of the strengths of the formulation (usually the highest strength unless a lower strength is chosen for reasons of safety); and

    v. in case of systemic availability - pharmacokinetics have been shown to be linear over the therapeutic dose range.

In vitro dissolution testing may also be suitable to confirm unchanged product quality and performance characteristics with minor formulation or manufacturing changes after approval.

3.2 When bioequivalence studies are not necessary

In following formulations and circumstances, bioequivalence between a new drug and the reference product may be considered self-evident with no further requirement for documentation:

a. When new drugs are to be administered parenterally (e.g., intravenous, intramuscular, subcutaneous, intrathecal administration etc.) as aqueous solutions and contain the same active substance(s) in the same concentration and the same excipients in comparable concentrations;

b. When the new drug is a solution for oral use, and contains the active substance in the same concentration, and does not contain an excipient that is known or suspected to affect gastro-intestinal transit or absorption of the active substance;

c. When the new drug is a gas;

d. When the new drug is a powder for reconstitution as a solution and the solution meets either criterion (a) or criterion (b) above;

e. When the new drug is an otic or ophthalmic or topical product prepared as aqueous solution and contains the same active substance(s) in the same concentration(s) and essentially the same excipients in comparable concentrations;

f. When the new drug is an inhalation product or a nasal spray, tested to be administered with or without essentially the same device as the reference product, prepared as aqueous solutions, and contain the same active substance(s) in the same concentration and essentially the same excipients in comparable concentrations. Special *in vitro* testing is required to document device performance comparison between reference inhalation product and the new drug product.

For (e) and (f) above, the applicant is expected to demonstrate that the excipients in the new drug are essentially the same and in comparable concentrations as those in the reference product. In the event this information about the reference product cannot be provided by the applicant, *in vivo* studies need to be performed.

4 DESIGN AND CONDUCT OF STUDIES

4.1 Pharmacokinetic Studies

4.1.1 Study Design

The basic design of an in-vivo bioavailability study is determined by the following:

I What is the scientific question(s) to be answered.

ii The nature of the reference material and the dosage form to be tested.

iii The availability of analytical methods.

iv Benefit-risk ratio considerations in regard to testing in humans.

The study should be designed in such a manner that the formulation effect can be distinguished from other effects. Typically, if two formulations are to be compared, a two-period, two-sequence crossover design is the design of choice with the two phases of treatment separated by an adequate washout period which should ideally be equal to or more than five half life's of the moieties to be measured.

Alternative study designs include the parallel design for very long half-life substances or the replicate design for substances with highly variable disposition.

Single-dose studies generally suffice. However situations as described below may demand a steady-state study design:

i Dose or time-dependant pharmacokinetics.

ii Some modified release products (in addition to single dose investigations)

iii Where problems of sensitivity preclude sufficiently precise plasma concentration measurements after single-dose administration.

iv If intra-individual variability in the plasma concentration or disposition precludes the possibility of demonstrating bioequivalence in a reasonably sized single-dose study and this variability is reduced at steady state.

4.1.2 Study Population

1. Selection of the Number of Subjects

The number of subjects required for a study should be statistically significant and is determined by the following considerations:

i The error variance associated with the primary characteristic to be studied as estimated from a pilot experiment, from previous studies or from published data.

ii The significance level desired: usually 0.05

iii The expected deviation from the reference product compatible with bioequivalence.

iv The required (discriminatory) power, normally 80% to detect the maximum allowable difference (usually 20%) in primary characteristics to be studied.

The number of subjects recruited should be sufficient to allow for possible withdrawals or removals (dropouts) from the study. It is acceptable to replace a subject withdrawn/drop out from the study once it has begun provided the substitute follows the same protocol originally intended for the withdrawn subject and he/she is tested under similar environmental and other controlled conditions.

However, the minimum number of subjects should not be less than 16 unless justified for ethical reasons.

Sequential or add-on studies are acceptable in specific cases e.g. where a large number of subjects are required or where the results of the study do not convey adequate statistical significance. In all cases the final statistical analysis must include data of all subjects or reasons for not including partial data as well as the un-included data must be documented in the final report.

2. Selection Criteria for Subjects

To minimize intra and inter individual variation subjects should be standardized as much as possible and acceptable. The studies should be normally performed on healthy adult volunteers with the aim to minimise variability and permit detection of differences between the study drugs. Subjects may be males or females; however the choice of gender should be consistent with usage and safety criteria.

Risks to women of childbearing potential should be considered on an individual basis. Women should be required to give assurance that they are neither pregnant, nor likely to become pregnant until after the study. This should be confirmed by a pregnancy test immediately prior to the first and last dose of the study. Women taking contraceptive drugs should normally not be included in the studies.

If the drug product is to be used predominantly in the elderly attempt should be made to include as many subjects of 60 years of age or older as possible. If the drug product is intended for use in both sexes attempt should be made to include similar proportions of males and females in the studies.

For a drug representing a potential hazard in one group of users, the choice of subjects may be narrowed, e.g., studies on teratogenic drugs should be conducted only on males.

For drugs primarily intended for use in only males or only females – volunteers of only respective gender should be included in the studies.

For drugs where the risk of toxicity or side effects is significant, studies may have to be carried out in patients with the concerned disease, but whose disease state is stable.

They should be screened for suitability by means of a comprehensive medical examination including clinical laboratory tests, an extensive review of medical history including medication history, use of oral contraceptives, alcohol intake, and smoking, use of drugs of abuse.

Depending on the study drugs therapeutic class and safety profile, special medical investigations may need to be carried out before, during and after the study.

3. Genetic Phenotyping

Phenotyping and/or genotyping of subjects should be considered for exploratory bioavailability studies and all studies using parallel group design. It may also be considered in crossover studies (e.g. bioequivalence, dose proportionality, food interaction studies etc.) for safety or pharmacokinetic reasons. If a drug is known to be subject to major genetic polymorphism, studies could be performed in panels of subjects of known phenotype or genotype for the polymorphism in question. While designing a study protocol, adequate care should be taken to consider Pharmacogenomic issues in the context of Indian population.

4.1.3 Study Conditions

Standardisation of the study environment, diet, fluid intake, post-dosing postures, exercise, sampling schedules etc. is important in all studies. Compliance to these standardisations should be stated in the protocol and reported at the end of the study, in order to reassure that all variability factors involved, except that of the products being tested, have been minimised. Unless the study design requires, subjects should abstain from smoking, drinking alcohol, coffee, tea, xanthine containing foods and beverages and fruit juices during the study and at least 48 hours before its commencement.

1. Selection of Blood Sampling Points/Schedules

The blood-sampling period in single-dose trials of an immediate release product should extend to at least three-elimination half-lives. Sampling should be continued for a sufficient period to ensure that the area extrapolated from the time of the last measured concentration to infinite time is only a small percentage (normally less than 20%) of the total AUC. The use of a truncated AUC is undesirable except in certain circumstances such as in the presence of enterohepatic recycling where the terminal elimination rate constant cannot be calculated accurately.

There should be at least three sampling points during the absorption phase, three to four at the projected Tmax, and four points during the elimination phase.

The number of points used to calculate the terminal elimination rate constant should be preferably determined by eye from a semi-logarithmic plot.

Intervals between successive data/sampling points used to calculate the terminal elimination rate constant should, in general, not be longer than the half-life of the study drug.

Where urinary excretion is measured in a single-dose study it is necessary to collect urine for seven or more half-lives.

2. Fasting and Fed State Considerations

Generally, a single dose study should be conducted after an overnight fast (at least 10 hours), with subsequent fast of 4 hours following dosing. For multiple dose fasting state studies, when an evening dose must be given, two hours of fasting before and after the dose is considered acceptable.

However, when it is recommended that the study drug be given with food (as would be in routine clinical practice), or where the dosage form is a modified release product, fed state studies need to be carried out in addition to the fasting state studies.

Fed state studies are also required when fasting state studies make assessment of C_{max} and T_{max} difficult.

Studies in the fed state require the consumption of a high-fat breakfast before dosing. Such a breakfast must be designed to provide 950 to 1000 KCals. At least 50% of these calories must come from fat, 15 to 20% from proteins and the rest from carbohydrates. The vast ethnic and cultural variations of the Indian subcontinent preclude the recommendation of any single standard high fat breakfast. Protocol should specify the suitable and appropriate diet. The high fat breakfast must be consumed approximately 15 minutes before dosing.

3. Steady State Studies

In following cases – an additional "steady state study" is considered appropriate:

i   Where the drug has a long terminal elimination half-life and blood concentrations after a single dose cannot be followed for a sufficient time.

ii   Where assay sensitivity is inadequate to follow the terminal elimination phase for an adequate period of time.

iii   For drugs, which are so toxic that ethically they should only be administered to patients for whom they are a necessary part of therapy, but where multiple dose therapy is required, e.g. many cytotoxics.

iv   For modified-release products where it is necessary to assess the fluctuation in plasma concentration over a dosage interval at steady state.

v   For those drugs which induce their own metabolism or show large intra individual variability.

vi   For enteric-coated preparations where the coating is innovative.

vii   For combination products where the ratio of plasma concentration of the individual drugs is important.

viii   For drugs that exhibit non-linear (i.e., dose- or time- dependent) pharmacokinetics.

ix   Where the drug is likely to accumulate in the body.

In steady state studies, the dosing schedule should follow the clinically recommended dosage regimen.

4.1.4 Characteristics to be investigated during bioavailability/ bioequivalence studies

In most cases evaluations of bioavailability and bioequivalence will be based upon the measured concentrations of the active drug substance(s) in the biological matrix. In some situations, however, the measurements of an active or inactive metabolite may be necessary. These situations include (a) where the concentrations of the drug(s) may be too low to accurately measure in the biological matrix, (b) limitations of the analytical method, (c) unstable drug(s), (d) drug(s) with a very short half-life or (e) in the case of prodrugs.

Racemates should be measured using an achiral assay method. Measurement of individual enantiomers in bioequivalence studies is recommended where all of the following criteria are met:

(a)   the enantiomers exhibit different pharmacodynamic characteristics

(b) the enantiomers exhibit different pharmacokinetic characteristics

(c) primary efficacy / safety activity resides with the minor enantiomer

(d) non-linear absorption is present for at least one of the enantiomers

The plasma-time concentration curve is mostly used to assess the rate and extent of absorption of the study drug. These include pharmacokinetic parameters such as the C_{max}, T_{max}, AUC_{0-t} and $AUC_{0-\tau}$.

For studies in the steady state $AUC_{0-\tau}$, C_{max}, C_{min} and degree of fluctuation should be calculated.

4.1.5 Bioanalytical Methodology

The bioanalytical methods used to determine the drug and/or its metabolites in plasma, serum, blood or urine or any other suitable matrix must be well characterised, standardised, fully validated and documented to yield reliable results that can be satisfactorily interpreted.

Although there are various stages in the development and validation of an analytical procedure, the validation of the analytical method can be envisaged to consist of two distinct phases:

1. The pre-study phase which comes before the actual start of the study and involves the validation of the method on biological matrix human plasma samples and spiked plasma samples.

2. The study phase in which the validated bioanalytical method is applied to the actual analysis of samples from bioavailability and bioequivalence studies mainly to confirm the stability, accuracy and precision.

1. Pre-study Phase

The following characteristics of the bioanalytical method must be evaluated and documented to ensure the acceptability of the performance and reliability of analytical results:

i.   Stability of the drug/metabolites in the biological matrix:

Stability of the drug and/or active metabolites in the biological matrix under the conditions of the experiment (including any period for which samples are stored before analyses) should be established. The stability data should also include the influence of at least three freezing and thawing cycles representative of actual sample handling. The absence of any sorption by the sampling containers and stoppers should also be established.

ii.   Specificity/Selectivity:

Data should be generated to demonstrate that the assay does not suffer from interference by endogenous compounds, degradation products, other drugs likely to be present in study samples, and metabolites of the drug(s) under study.

iii   Sensitivity:

Sensitivity is the capacity of the test procedure to record small variations in concentration. The analytical method chosen should be capable of assaying the drug/metabolites over the expected concentration range. A reliable lowest limit of quantification should be established based on an intra- and inter-day coefficient of variation usually not greater than 20 percent. The limit of detection (the lowest concentration that can be differentiated from background levels) is usually lower than the limit of quantification. Values between limit of quantification and limit of detection should be identified as "Below Quantification Limits."

iv. Precision and Accuracy:

Precision (the degree of reproducibility of individual assays) should be established by replicate assays on standards, preferably at several concentrations. Accuracy is the degree to which the 'true' value of the concentration of drug is estimated by the assay. Precision and accuracy should normally be documented at three concentrations (low, medium, high) where 'low' is in the vicinity of the lowest concentration to be measured, 'high' is a value in the vicinity of Cmax and 'medium' is a suitable intermediate value.

Intra-assay precision (within days) in terms of coefficient of variation should be no more than 15%, although no more than 20% may be more realistic at values near the lower limit of quantification. Inter-assay precision (between days) may be higher than 15% but not more than 20%.

Accuracy can be assessed in conjunction with precision and is a measure of the extent to which measured concentrations deviate from true or nominal concentrations of analytical standards. In general, an accuracy of ±15% should be attained.

v. Recovery:

Documentation of extraction recovery at high, medium and low concentrations is essential since methods with low recovery are, in general, more prone to inconsistency. If recovery is low, alternative methods should be investigated. Recovery of any internal standard used should also be assessed.

vi. Range and linearity:

The quantitative relationship between concentration and response should be adequately characterized over the entire range of expected sample concentrations. For linear relationships, a standard curve should be defined by at least five concentrations. If the concentration response function is non-linear, additional points would be necessary to define the non-linear portions of the curve. Extrapolation beyond the standard curve is not acceptable.

Vii Analytical System Stability:

To assure that the analytical system remains stable over the time course of the assay, the reproducibility of the standard curve should be monitored during the assay. A minimal design would be to run analytical standards at the beginning and at the end of the analytical run.

2. Study Phase

In general, with acceptable variability as defined by validation data, the analysis of biological sample can be done by single determination without a need for a duplicate or replicate analysis. The need for duplicate analysis should be assessed on a case-by-case basis. A procedure should be developed that documents the reason for re-analysis.

A standard curve should be generated for each analytical run for each analyte and should be used to calculate the concentration of the analyte in the unknown samples assayed with that run. It is important to use a standard curve that will cover the entire range of concentrations in the unknown samples. Estimation of unknowns by extrapolations of standard curves below the lowest standard concentration or above the highest standard concentration is not recommended. Instead, it is suggested that standard curve should be redetermined or sample should be re-assayed after dilution. Quality control sample should be used to accept or reject the run.

3. Quality Control Samples:

Quality control samples are samples with known concentration prepared by spiking drug-free biological fluid with drug. These samples should be prepared in low, medium and high concentration. To avoid possible confusion between quality control samples and standard solutions during the review process, preparation of quality control samples at concentrations different from those used for the calibration is recommended. For stable analytes, quality control samples should be prepared in the fluid of interest at the time of pre-study assay validation or at the time of study sample collection, and stored with the study samples. For less stable analytes, daily or weekly quality control samples may have to be prepared.

A quality control sample for each concentration should be assayed on each occasion that study samples are assayed, and the concentration determined by reference to that day's calibration standards. If the concentration values determined for the controls are not within ±15% of the expected concentrations, the batch should be considered for re-analysis.

4. Repeat Analysis:

In most studies some samples will require re-analysis because of aberrant results due to processing errors, equipment failure or poor chromatography. The reasons for re-analysis of such samples should be stated. The criteria for repeat analyses should be determined prior to running the study and recorded in the protocol / laboratory standard operating procedures.

4.1.6 Statistical Evaluation

1. Data analysis:

The primary concern in bio-equivalence assessment is to limit the consumer's risk i.e., erroneously accepting bioequivalence and also at the same time minimizing the manufacture's risk i.e., erroneously rejecting bioequivalence. This is done by using appropriate statistical methods for data analysis and adequate sample size.

2. Statistical analysis:

The statistical procedure should be specified in the protocol itself. In case of bioequivalence studies the procedures should lead to a decision scheme which is symmetrical with respect to the two formulations (i.e. leading to the same decision whether the new formulation is compared to the reference product or the reference product to the new formulation).

The statistical analysis (e.g. ANOVA) should take into account sources of variation that can be reasonably assumed to have an effect on the response.

The 90% confidence interval for the ratio of the population means (Test/reference) or two one sided-t tests with the null hypothesis of nonbioequivalence at the 5% significance level for the parameter under consideration are considered for testing bioequivalence.

To meet the assumption of normality of data underlying the statistical analysis, the logarithmic transformation should be carried out for the pharmacokinetic parameters Cmax and AUC before performing statistical analysis. However, it is recommended not to verify the assumptions underlying the statistical analysis before making logarithmic transformation.

The analysis of T_{max} is desirable if it is clinically relevant. The parameter T_{max} should be analysed using non-parametric methods. In addition to above, summary statistics such as minimum, maximum and ratio should be given.

3. Criteria for bioequivalence:

To establish Bioequivalence, the calculated 90% confidence interval for AUC and Cmax should fall within the bioequivalence range, usually 80-125%. This is equivalent to the rejection of two one sided-t tests with the null hypothesis of nonbioequivalence at 5% level of significance. The non-parametric 90% confidence interval for Tmax should lie within a clinically acceptable range.

Tighter limits for permissible differences in bioavailability may be required for drugs that have:

    i   A narrow therapeutic index.

    Ii   A serious, dose-related toxicity.

    Iii   A steep dose/effect curve, or

    iv   A non-linear pharmacokinetics within the therapeutic dose range.

A wider acceptance range may be acceptable if it is based on sound clinical justification.

In case of supra-bioavailability, a reformulation followed by a fresh bioequivalence study will be necessary. Otherwise, clinical trial data on new formulation will be required to support the application, especially dosage recommendations. Such formulations are usually not be accepted as therapeutically equivalent to the existing reference product. The name of the new product should preclude confusion with the earlier approved product.

4. Deviations from the study plan

The method of analysis should be defined in the protocol. The protocol should specify methods for handling drop-outs and for identifying biologically implausible outliers. Post hoc exclusion of outliers is not recommended. A scientific explanation should be provided to justify the exclusion of a volunteer from the analysis.

4.1.7 Special considerations for Modified-Release Drug Products

For the purpose of these guidelines modified release products include:

i   delayed release

ii   sustained release

iii   mixed immediate and sustained release

iv   mixed delayed and sustained release

v   mixed immediate and delayed release

Generally, these products should:

i   act as modified-release formulations and meet the label claim

ii   preclude the possibility of any dose dumping effect

iii   there must be a significant difference between the performance of modified release product and the conventional release product when used as reference product.

iv   provide a therapeutic performance comparable to the reference immediate release formulation administered by the same route in multiple doses (of an equivalent daily amount) or to the reference modified-release formulation;

v   produce consistent pharmacokinetic performance between individual dosage units; and

vi   produce plasma levels which lie within the therapeutic range (where appropriate) for the proposed dosing intervals at steady state.

If all of the above conditions are not met but the applicant considers the formulation to be acceptable, justification to this effect should be provided.

i. Study Parameters

Bioavailability data should be obtained for all modified release drug products although the type of studies required and the pharmacokinetic parameters which should be evaluated may differ depending on the active ingredient involved. Factors to be considered include whether or not the formulation represents the first market entry of the drug substance, and the extent of accumulation of the drug after repeated dosing.

If the formulation is the first market entry of the drug substance, the product's pharmacokinetic parameters should be determined. If the formulation is a second or subsequent market entry then comparative bioavailability studies using an appropriate reference product should be performed.

ii. Study design

Study design will be single dose or single and multiple dose based on the modified release products that are likely to accumulate or unlikely to accumulate both in the fasted and non-fasting state. If the effect of food on the reference product is not known (or it is known that food affects its absorption), two separate two-way cross-over studies, one in the fasted state and the other in the fed state, may be carried out. If it is known with certainty (e.g. from published data) that the reference product is not affected by food, then a three-way cross-over study may be appropriate with:

a. the reference product in the fasting state

b. the test product in the fasted state, and

c. the test product in the fed state.

iii. Requirements for modified release formulations unlikely to accumulate

This section outlines the requirements for modified release formulations which are used at a dose interval that is not likely to lead to accumulation in the body ($AUC0-$ /$AUC0-$ 0.8).

When the modified release product is the first market entry of that type of dosage form, the reference product should normally be the innovator's immediate release formulation. The comparison should be between a single dose of the modified release formulation and doses of the immediate-release formulation which it is intended to replace. The latter must be administered according to the established dosing regimen.

When the modified release product is the second or subsequent entry on the market, comparison should be with the reference modified release product for which bioequivalence is claimed.

Studies should be performed with single dose administration in the fasting state as well as following an appropriate meal at a specified time.

The following pharmacokinetic parameters should be calculated from plasma (or relevant biological matrix) concentrations of the drug and/or major metabolite(s):

$AUC_{0-\tau}$, AUC_{0-t}, $AUC_{0-\infty}$, C_{max} (where the comparison is with an existing modified release product), and k_{el}

The 90% confidence interval calculated using log transformed data for the ratios (Test: Reference) of the geometric mean AUC (for both AUC_{0-} and AUC_{0-t}) and C_{max} (where the comparison is with an existing modified release product) should generally be within the range 80 to 125% both in the fasting state and following the administration of an appropriate meal at a specified time before taking the drug.

The pharmacokinetic parameters should support the claimed dose delivery attributes of the modified-release dosage form.

iv. Requirements for modified release formulations likely to accumulate

This section outlines the requirements for modified release formulations that are used at dose intervals that are likely to lead to accumulation ($AUC_{0-\tau}/AUC_{0-\infty} < 0.8$).

When a modified release product is the first market entry of the modified release type, the reference formulation is normally the innovator's immediate-release formulation. Both a single dose and steady state doses of the modified release formulation should be compared with doses of the immediate-release formulation which it is intended to replace. The immediate-release product should be administered according to the conventional dosing regimen.

Studies should be performed with single dose administration in the fasting state as well as following an appropriate meal. In addition, studies are required at steady state. The following pharmacokinetic parameters should be calculated from single dose studies: $AUC_{0-\tau}$, AUC_{0-t}, $AUC_{0-\infty}$, C_{max} (where the comparison is with an existing modified release product), and kel. The following parameters should be calculated from steady state studies: $AUC_{0-\tau(ss)}$, C_{max}, C_{min}, C_{pd} and degree of fluctuation.

When the modified release product is the second or subsequent modified release entry, single dose and steady state comparisons should normally be made with the reference modified release product for which bioequivalence is claimed.

The 90% confidence interval for the ratio of geometric means (Test: Reference drug) of AUC (for both AUC_{0-} and AUC_{0-t}) and Cmax (where the comparison is with an existing modified release product) determined using log-transformed data should generally be within the range 80 to 125% when the products are compared after single dose administration in both the fasting state and the fed state.

The 90% confidence interval for the ratio of geometric means (Test: Reference drug) for $AUC_{0- (ss)}$, Cmax, and Cmin determined using log-transformed data should generally be within the range 80 to 125% when the formulations are compared at steady state.

The pharmacokinetic parameters should support the claimed attributes of the modified-release dosage form.

Pharmacodynamic data may reinforce or clarify interpretation of differences in the plasma concentration data.

Where these studies do not show bioequivalence, comparative efficacy and safety data may be required for the new product.

4.2 Pharmacodynamic Studies

Studies in healthy volunteers or patients using pharmacodynamic parameters may be used for establishing equivalence between two pharmaceutical products. These studies may become necessary if quantitative analysis of the drug and/or metabolite(s) in plasma or urine cannot be made with sufficient accuracy and sensitivity. Furthermore, pharmacodynamic studies in humans are required if measurements of drug concentrations cannot be used as surrogate endpoints for the demonstration of efficacy and safety of the particular pharmaceutical product e.g., for topical products without an intended absorption of the drug into the systemic circulation.

In case, only pharmacodynamic data is collected and provided, the applicant should outline what other methods were tried and why they were found unsuitable.

The following requirements should be recognised when planning, conducting and assessing the results from a pharmacodynamic study:

i   The response measured should be a pharmacological or therapeutic effect which is relevant to the claims of efficacy and/or safety of the drug.

ii   The methodology adopted for carrying out the study should be validated for precision, accuracy, reproducibility and specificity.

iii   Neither the test nor the reference product should produce a maximal response in the course of the study, since it may be impossible to distinguish differences between formulations given in doses that produce such maximal responses. Investigation of dose-response relationship may become necessary.

iv   The response should be measured quantitatively under double-blind conditions and be recorded in a instrument-produced or instrument recorded fashion on a repetitive basis to provide a record of pharmacodynamic events which are a substitute for plasma concentrations.

   If such measurements are not possible, recordings on visual-analog scales may be used. In instances, where data are limited to qualitative (categorized) measurements, appropriate special statistical analyses will be required.

v   Non-responders should be excluded from the study by prior screening. The criteria by which responders *versus* non-responders are identified must be stated in the protocol.

vi   Where an important placebo effect can occur, comparison between products can only be made by a priori consideration of the placebo effect in the study design. This may be achieved by adding a third period/phase with placebo treatment, in the design of the study.

vii   A crossover or parallel study design should be used, as appropriate.

viii   When pharmacodynamic studies are to be carried out on patients, the underlying pathology and natural history of the condition should be considered in the study design. There should be knowledge of the reproducibility of the base-line conditions.

ix   In studies where continuous variables could be recorded, the time course of the intensity of the drug action can be described in the same way as in a study where plasma concentrations are measured. From this, parameters can be derived which describe the area under the effect-time curve, the maximum response and the time when the maximum response occurred.

x   Statistical considerations for the assessments of the outcomes are in principle, the same as in pharmacokinetic studies.

xi   A correction for the potential non-linearity of the relationship between dose and area under the effect-time curve should be made on the basis of the outcome of the dose ranging study.

The conventional acceptance range as applicable to pharmacokinetic studies and bioequivalence is not appropriate (too large) in most cases. This range should therefore be defined in the protocol on a case-to-case basis.

4.3   Comparative Clinical Studies

In several instances (For example, section 3.1.1(e) above), the plasma concentration time-profile data may not be suitable to assess equivalence between two formulations. Whereas in some of the cases pharmacodynamic studies can be an appropriate tool for establishing equivalence, in other instances this type of study cannot be performed because of lack of meaningful pharmacodynamic parameters which can be measured and a comparative clinical study has to be performed in order to demonstrate equivalence between two formulations. Comparative clinical studies may also be required to be carried out for certain orally administered drug products when pharmacokinetic and pharmacodynamic studies are not feasible. However, in such cases, the applicant should outline what other methods were tried and why they were found unsuitable.

If a clinical study is considered as being undertaken to prove equivalence, the appropriate statistical principles should be applied to demonstrate bioequivalence. The number of patients to be included in the study will depend on the variability of the target parameters and the acceptance range, and is usually much higher than the number of subjects in bioequivalence studies.

The following items are important and need to be defined in the protocol in advance:

a. The target parameters which usually represent relevant clinical end-points from which the intensity and the onset, if applicable and relevant, of the response are to be derived.

b. The size of the acceptance range has to be defined case-to- case taking into consideration the specific clinical conditions. These include, among others, the natural course of the disease, the efficacy of available treatments and the chosen target parameter. In contrast to bioequivalence studies (where a conventional acceptance range is applied) the size of the acceptance range in clinical trials cannot be based on a general consensus on all the therapeutic classes and indications.

c. The presently used statistical method is the confidence interval approach. The main concern is to rule out that the test product is inferior to the reference product by more than the specified amount. Hence, a one-sided confidence interval (for efficacy and/or safety) may be appropriate. The confidence intervals can be derived from either parametric or nonparametric methods.

d. Where appropriate, a placebo leg should be included in the design.

e. In some cases, it is relevant to include safety end-points in the final comparative assessments.

4.4   *In Vitro Studies*

In certain situations a comparative *in vitro* dissolution study may be sufficient to demonstrate equivalence between two drug products (See Section 3).

The test methodology adopted should be in line with the pharmacopoeial requirements unless those requirements are shown to be unsatisfactory. Alternative methods may be acceptable provided they have sufficient discriminatory power.

Dissolution studies should generally be carried out under mild agitation conditions at 37±0.5°C and at physiologically relevant pH. More than one batch of each formulation should be tested. Comparative dissolution profiles, rather than single point dissolution test data, should be generated. The design should include:

i   Individually testing of at least twelve dosage units (e.g., tablets, capsules) of each batch. Mean and individual results should be reported along with their standard deviations or standard errors.

ii Measuring the percentage of nominal content released at a number of suitably spaced time points to provide a profile for each batch, e.g. at 10, 20 and 30 minutes or as appropriate to achieve virtually complete dissolution.

iii Determining the dissolution profile in at least three aqueous media covering the pH range of 1.0 to 6.8 or in cases where considered necessary, pH range of 1.0 to 8.0.

iv Conducting the tests on each batch using the same apparatus and, if possible, on the same or consecutive days.

Comparisons of the dissolution profiles may be made by any of the established model-independent or model-dependent methods.

5. DOCUMENTATION

With respect to the conduct of bioequivalence/bioavailability studies following important documents must be maintained:

i. Clinical Data:

    a. All relevant documents as required to be maintained for compliance with GCP Guidelines

ii. Details of the analytical method validation including the following:

    a. System suitability test

    b. Linearity range

    c. Lowest limit of quantitation

    d. QC sample analysis

    e. Stability sample analysis

    f. Recovery experiment result

iii. Analytical data of volunteer plasma samples which should include the following:

    a. Validation data of analytical methods used

    b. Chromatograms of all volunteers, including any aberrant chromatograms

    c. Inter-day and intra-day variation of assay results

    d. Details including chromatograms of any repeat analysis performed

    e. Calibration status of the instruments

iv. Raw data

v. All comments of the chief investigator regarding the data of the study submitted for review.

vi. A copy of the final report

STUDY REPORT

The bioequivalence or bioavailability report should give the complete documentation of its protocol, conduct and evaluation.

The report should include (as a minimum) the following information:

a. Table of contents

b. Title of the study

c. Names and credentials of responsible investigators

d. Signatures of the principal and other responsible investigators authenticating their respective sections of the report

e. Site of the study and facilities used

f. The period of dates over which the clinical and analytical steps were conducted

g. Names and batch numbers of the products compared

h. A signed declaration that this was identical to that intended for marketing.

i. Results of assays and other pharmaceutical tests (e.g., physical description, dimensions, mean weight, weight uniformity, comparative dissolution) carried out on the batches of products compared

j. Full protocol for the study including a copy of the ICF and criteria for inclusion/exclusion or withdrawal of subjects

k. Report of protocol deviations, violations

l. Documentary evidence that the study was approved by an independent ethics committee and was carried out in accordance with GCP/GLP.

m. Demographic data of subjects

n. Names and addresses of subjects

o. Details of and justifications for protocol deviations

p. Details of dropout and withdrawals from the study should be fully documented and accounted for

q. Details of analytical methods used, full validation data, quality control data and criteria for accepting or rejecting assay results

r. Representative chromatograms covering the whole concentration range for all, standard and quality control samples as well as specimens analysed

s. Sampling schedules and deviations of the actual times from the scheduled

t. Details of how pharmacokinetic parameters were calculated

u. Documentation related to statistical analysis:

  i. Randomization schedule

  ii. Volunteer wise plasma concentration and time points for test and reference products

  iii. Volunteer wise AUC_{0-t}, $AUC_{0-\infty}$, C_{max}, T_{max}, K_{el}, and $t_{1/2}$ for test and reference products

  iv. Logarithmic transformed measures used for BE demonstration

  v. ANOVA for AUC_{0-t}, $AUC_{0-\infty}$, C_{max}

  vi. Inter-subject, intra-subject and/or total variability if possible

  vii. Confidence intervals for AUC_{0-t}, AUC_{0-}, Cmax (Confidence interval (CI) values should not be rounded off; therefore, to pass a CI range of 80 to 125, the values should be at least 80.00 and not more than 125.00

  viii. Geometric mean, arithmetic mean, ratio of means for AUC_{0-t}, $AUC_{0-\infty}$, C_{max}

  ix. Partial AUC, only if it is used

  x. C_{min}, C_{max}, C_{pd}, $AUC_{0-\tau}$, degree of fluctuation $[(C_{max} - C_{min})/C_{av}]$ and swing $[(C_{max} - C_{min})/C_{min}]$, if steady state studies are employed.

6. FACILITIES FOR CONDUCTING BIOAVAILABILITY AND/OR BIOEQUIVALENCE STUDIES

6.1 Legal identity

The organization, conducting the bioequivalence / bioavailability studies, or the parent organization to which it belongs, must be a legally constituted body with appropriate statutory registrations.

6.2 Impartiality, confidentiality, independence and integrity:

The organization shall:

a. have managerial staff with the authority and the resources needed to discharge their duties.

b. have arrangements to ensure that its personnel are free from any commercial, financial and other pressures which might adversely affect the quality of their work.

c. be organized in such a way that confidence in its independence of judgment and integrity is maintained at all times.

d. have documented policies and procedures, where relevant, to ensure the protection of its sponsors' confidential information and proprietary rights.

e. not engage in any activity that may jeopardize the trust in its independence of judgement and integrity

f. have documented policies and procedures for the safety of human rights and the use of human subjects in research consistent with Schedule Y (refer Drugs & Cosmetics Act and Rules) and GCP Guidelines

g. have documented policies and procedures for scientific integrity including procedures dealing with and reporting possible scientific misconduct.

6.3   Organisation and Management

The study site organization must include the following:

a. An Investigator who has the overall responsibility to provide of the human subjects. The Investigator(s) should possess appropriate medical qualifications and relevant experience for conducting pharmacokinetic studies.

b. The site should have identified adequately qualified and trained personnel to perform the following functions:

   i   Clinical Pharmacological Unit (CPU) management

   ii   Analytical laboratory management

   iii   Data handling and interpretation

   iv   Documentation and report preparation

   v   Quality assurance of all operations in the centre

6.4   Documented Standard Operating Procedures

The center shall establish and maintain a quality system appropriate to the type, range and volume of its activities. All operations at the site must be conducted as per the authorized and documented standard operating procedures. These documented procedures should be available to the respective personnel for ready reference. The procedures covered must include those that ensure compliance with all aspects of:

a. GCP Guidelines

b. Good laboratory practice guidelines issued by Ministry of Health & Family Welfare

A partial list of procedures for which documented standard operating procedures should be available includes:

a. maintenance of working standards (pure substances) and respective documentation.

b. withdrawal, storage and handling of biological samples.

c. maintenance, calibration and validation of instruments.

d. managing medical as well as non-medical emergency situations

e. handling of biological fluids

f. managing laboratory hazards

g. disposal procedures for clinical samples and laboratory wastes

h. documentation of clinical pharmacology unit observations, volunteer data and analytical data

i. obtaining informed consent from volunteers

j. volunteer screening and recruitment and management of ineligible volunteers

k. volunteer recycling (using the same volunteer for more than one study

l. randomization code management

m. study subject management at the site (including check-in and check-out procedures)

n. recording and reporting protocol deviations

o. recording, reporting and managing scientific misconduct

p. monitoring and quality assurance

Wherever possible, disposable (sterile, wherever applicable) medical devices must be used for making subject interventions.

If services of a laboratory or a facility other than those available at the site (whether with in India or outside the country) are to be availed – its/their name(s), address(s) and specific services to be used should be documented.

6.5   Clinical Pharmacological Unit

It must have adequate space and facilities to house at least 16 volunteers. Adequate area must be provided for dining and recreation of volunteers, separate from their sleeping area.

Additional space and facilities should also be provided for the following:

a. Office and administrative functions

b. Sample collection and storage

c. Control sample storage

d. Wet chemical laboratory

e. Instrumental Laboratory

f. Library

g. Documentation archival room

h. Facility for washing, cleaning and Toilets

i. Microbiological laboratory (Optional)

j. Radio Immuno – Assay room (optional)

7. MAINTENANCE OF RECORDS OF BA/BE STUDIES

All records of in vivo or in vitro tests conducted on any marketed batch of a drug product to assure that the product meets a bioequivalence requirement shall be maintained by the Sponsor for at least 2 years after the expiration date of the batch and submitted to CDSCO on request.

8. RETENTION OF BA/BE SAMPLES

All samples of test and reference drug products used in bioavailability / bioequivalence study should be retained by the organization carrying out the bioavailability / bioequivalence study for a period of three years after the conduct of the study or one year after the expiry of the drug, whichever is earlier. The study sponsor and/or drug manufacturer should provide to the testing facility batches of the test and reference drug products in such a manner that the reserve samples can be selected randomly. This is to ensure that the samples are in fact representative of the batches provided by the study sponsor and/or drug manufacturer and that they are retained in their original containers. Each reserve sample should consist of a quantity sufficient to carry out twice all the *in-vitro* and *in-vivo* tests required during bioavailability / bioequivalence study.

The reserve sample should be stored under conditions consistent with product labelling and in an area segregated from the area where testing is conducted and with access limited to authorized personnel.

9. SPECIAL TOPICS

9.1   Food effect bioavailability studies

Food effect study is required when there is a possibility to have effect of food on the bioavailability of the drug. Food effect bioavailability studies focus on effects of food on the release of the drug substance from the drug product as well as the absorption of the drug substance. Usually, a single dose crossover study is recommended for BA and BE studies.

9.2   Long Half-life Drugs

For BE determination of an oral product with long half life, a single dose crossover study can be conducted, provided an adequate wash out period is used. If due to longer periods, chances of drop outs as well as intra subject variation are higher with routine cross over designs; parallel group designs can be used. In all cases, blood sampling period should be adequate to describe the plasma concentration time profile. Cmax and a suitably truncated AUC can be used to characterize peak and total drug exposure, respectively. For drugs, demonstrating high intra-subject variability in distribution and clearance, AUC truncation warrants caution. In such cases, sponsors and/or applicants should consult the regulatory authority.

9.3   Early Exposure

In general, bioequivalence may be demonstrated by measurements of peak and total exposure for an immediate release product. However, in situations such as rapid onset of an analgesic effect or to avoid an excessive hypotensive action of an antihypertensive, an early exposure measure may be informative on the basis of appropriate clinical efficacy/safety trials and/or pharmacokinetic / pharmacodynamic studies that call for better control of drug absorption into the systemic circulation. In these situations, use of partial AUC is recommended as an early exposure measure. The partial area should be truncated at Tmax values for the reference formulation. At least two quantifiable samples should be collected before the expected peak time to allow adequate estimation of the partial area.

Individual and Population Bioequivalence

The current practice of evaluating bioequivalence has been termed as average bioequivalence. Whereas in individual bioequivalence, determination of the intra subject variation of drug response is important. By "population bioequivalence" we mean a bioequivalence criterion that requires the distribution of the formulation to be sufficiently similar to that of the reference in some appropriate population. Average bioequivalence is a special case of population bioequivalence.

The average bioequivalence of the two formulations is important in the case of prescribability. However, Individual bioequivalence is required in case of switchability.

Assessment of individual bioequivalence is an interesting and exciting alternative to the current practice of evaluating average bioequivalence. The evaluation of individual bioequivalence requires values of intra-subject variability of the test and reference formulations. Hence the assessment of individual bioequivalence is done based on three or four period designs. Replicate study designs provide such information.

Up till now, bioequivalence studies are designed to evaluate average bioequivalence. Experience with population and individual bioequivalence studies is limited. Hence no specific recommendation is proposed on this matter. However, for highly variable drugs, individual bioequivalence can be considered.

MINISTRY OF HEALTH AND FAMILY WELFARE

(Department of Health and Family Welfare)

NOTIFICATION

New Delhi, the 3rd April, 2017

G.S.R. 327(E).—Whereas the draft of certain rules further to amend the Drugs and Cosmetics Rules, 1945 was published as required by sections 12 and 33 of the Drugs and Cosmetics Act, 1940 (23 of 1940) in the Gazette of India, Extraordinary, Part II, Section 3, Sub-section (i), dated the 2nd February, 2017 vide notification of the Government of India in the Ministry of Health and Family Welfare, number G.S.R. 102(E), dated the 2nd February, 2017 for inviting objections and suggestions from all persons likely to be affected thereby before the expiry of a period of forty-five days from the date on which copies of the Official Gazette containing the said notification was made available to the public;

And whereas the copies of the said Gazette were made available to the public on 2nd February, 2017;

And, whereas, objections and suggestions received from the public on the said rules have been considered by the Central Government.

Now, therefore, in exercise of the powers conferred by sections 12 and 33 of the said Act, the Central Government, after consultation with the Drugs Technical Advisory Board, hereby makes the following rules further to amend the Drugs and Cosmetics Rules, 1945, namely:-

1. These rules may be called Drugs and Cosmetics (Ninth Amendment) Rules, 2017.

(2) They shall come into force on the date of their publication in the Official Gazette.

2. In the Drugs and Cosmetics Rules, 1945 (hereinafter referred to as the said rules), in rule 2, after clause (a), following shall be inserted, namely:-

(aa) "biopharmaceutical classification system" means a system used to classify drugs on the basis of solubility and permeability, classified as category I- high solubility and high permeability, category II- low solubility and high permeability, category III- high solubility and low permeability, and category IV- low solubility and low permeability.";

3. In the said rules, in rule 74, after clause (p), the following clause shall inserted, namely.-

"(q) the applicant shall submit the result of bioequivalence study referred to in Schedule Y, along with the application for grant of a licence of oral dosage form of drugs specified under category II and category IV of the biopharmaceutical classification system.".

4. In the said rules, in rule 74B, after clause (7), the following clause shall inserted, namely.-

"(8) the applicant shall submit the result of bioequivalence study referred to in Schedule Y, along with the application for grant of a licence of oral dosage form of drugs specified under category II and category IV of the biopharmaceutical classification system.".

5. In the said rules, in rule 76, after clause (9), the following clause shall inserted, namely.-

"(10) the applicant shall submit the result of bioequivalence study referred to in Schedule Y, along with the application for grant of a licence of oral dosage form of drugs specified under category II and category IV of the biopharmaceutical classification system.".

6. In the said rules, in rule 78, after clause (q), the following clause shall inserted, namely.-

"(r) the applicant shall submit the result of bioequivalence study referred to in Schedule Y, along with the application for grant of a licence of oral dosage form of drugs specified under category II and category IV of the biopharmaceutical classification system.".

7. In the said rules, in rule 78A, after clause (8), the following clause shall inserted, namely.-

"(9) the applicant shall submit the result of bioequivalence study referred to in Schedule Y, along with the application for grant of a licence of oral dosage form of drugs specified under category II and category IV of the biopharmaceutical classification system.".

[F. No. X.11014/12/2016-DRS]

K. L. SHARMA, Jt. Secy.

Foot note: Principal rules were published in the Official Gazette vide notification number F.28-10/45-H (1), dated the 21st December, 1945 and last amended vide notification number G.S.R. 303 (E) dated the 30th March, 2017.

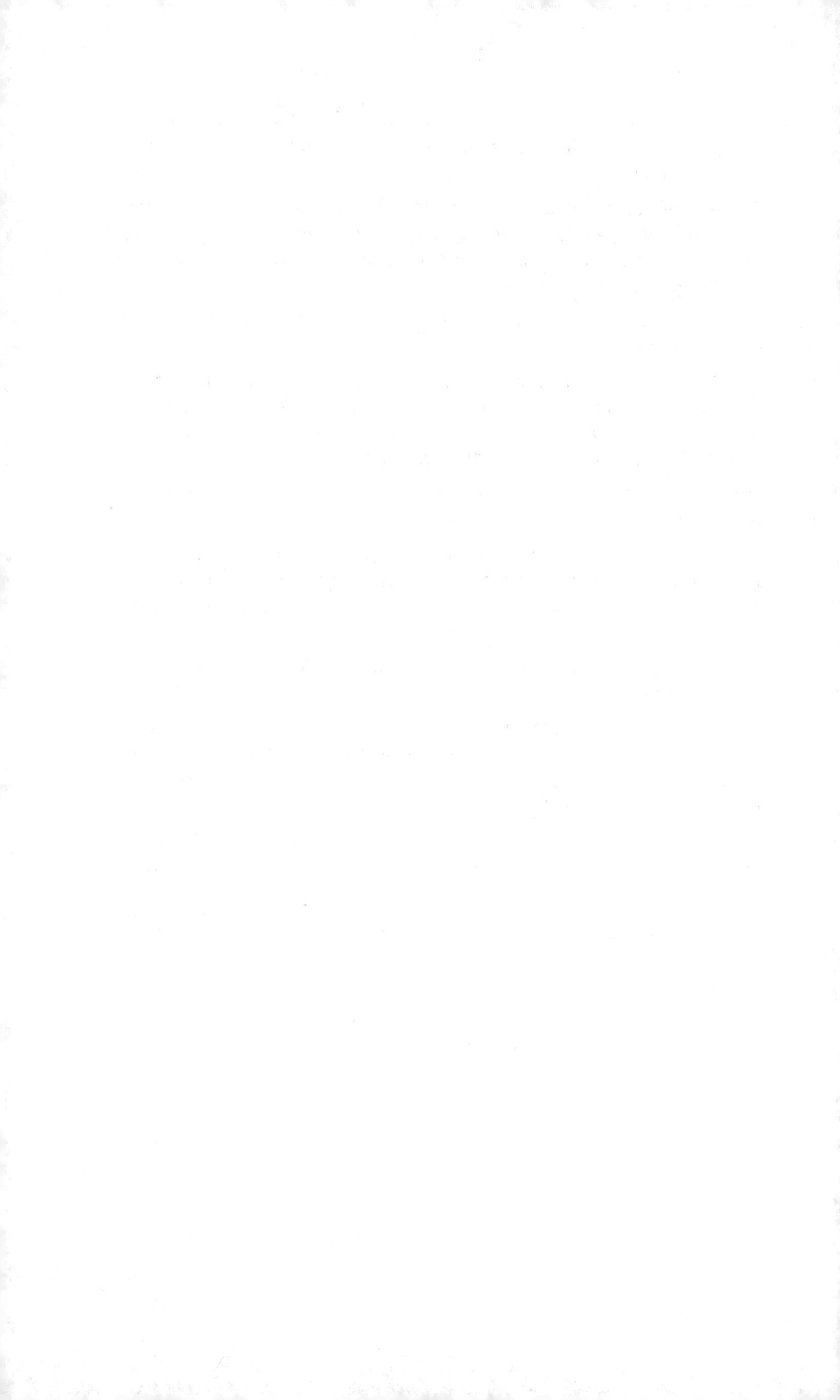

About the Authors

Dr. Bhaswati Pal
MBA, Ph. D

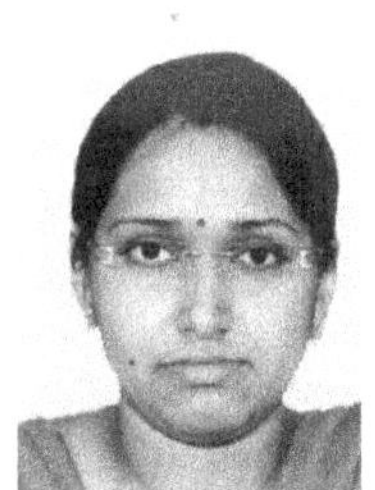

Dr. Pal had completed her Bachelor in Business Administration in HR studies from West Bengal University of Technology and Masters in Business Administration & Doctorate in Clinical Research from Indian School of Business Management, Mumbai under Stamford University, Hong Kong in 2012 and 2018 respectively.

She has experience in medical documentation, bioequivalence Study, Drug Archiving in healthcare Sector. Her thesis titled "Management and Regulatory aspects to establish a CRO for conducting BA/BE Study" awarded as "Award of Excellence" by panel of co-professors of Indian School of Business Management, Mumbai. She had actively participated in eight Good Clinical Practices Training conducted by Prof. Dr. Suparna Chatterjee, M.D, IPGME & R, Kolkata & Dr. Supriyo Choudhury, MD, Assistant Professor, Sagar Dutta Medical College from 2011 to 2018.

Since 2009 she had been working with TAAB Biostudy Services, as a Senior Executive &Team Leader, HR. Presently she is one of the Managing Partners of TAAB Biostudy Services.

Dr. Shubhasis Dan,
M. Pharm, Ph. D

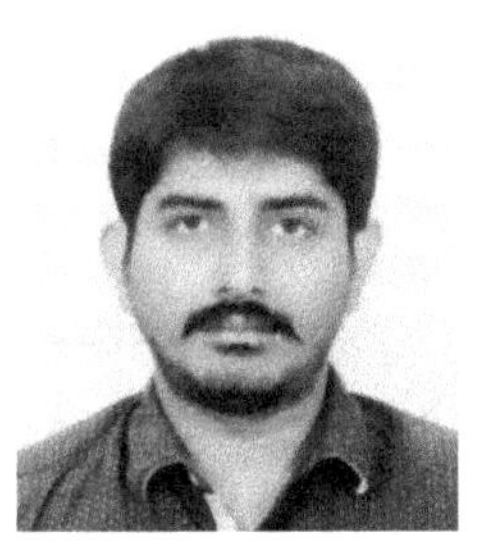

Dr. Dan joined as a Research Scholar (initially Fellow, DST, New Delhi & later UGC-BSR Meritorious Fellow) in the Bioequivalence Study Centre, Dept. of Pharmaceutical Technology, Jadavpur University. Being a pharma post graduate (M. Pharm), he completed his doctoral research under the guidance of Prof. T K Pal and awarded in Ph. D from Jadavpur University in 2017.

He is working with a CRO (CDSCO approved BA/BE Study Centre) since 2011, which results in better understanding of clinical regulatory as well as its implementations inside of the organization towards ensuring the smooth functioning.

Dr. Dan is presently associated with TAAB Biostudy Services, Kolkata (CDSCO approved BA/BE Study Centre) as a Team Leader, Clinical Studies and Regulatory Affairs with an obligation to interact with disciplinary groups from the Sponsor (different pharma companies), Regulators as well as Ethics Committee personals. Besides, he is similarly engaged in the preparation of protocol, SOP, dossiers and reviewing reports to satisfy the requirements of other regulatory bodies like ISO, NABL etc which ensures Dr. Dan's competence with the CDSCO policies and regulations related to clinical research.

Without ignoring the commercial responsibilities, efforts were made by Dr. Dan to endorse the academic activities through national and international publications (more than 30) related to formulation development, analytical and bio-analytical method development and validation of drugs in human plasma, regulatory reviews etc, which help to spread the goodwill of the associated institutions.

Prof. (Dr.) Tapan Kumar Pal,
M. Che (Gold Medalist), F.I.E, VDI (Germany)

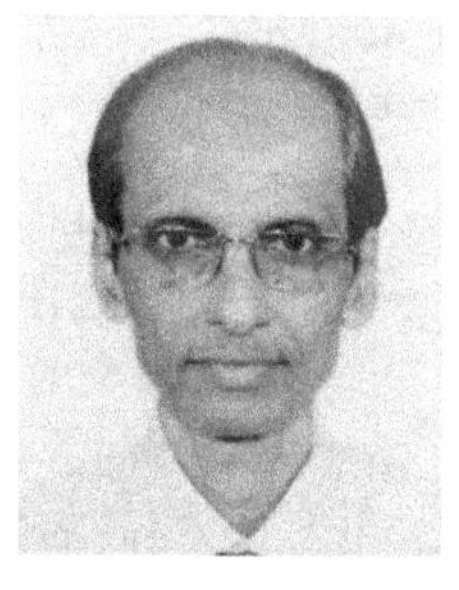

Prof. Dr. Tapan Kumar Pal, Former Professor and HOD, Department of Pharmaceutical Technology, Jadavpur University is now attached to the same university as Emeritus Medical Scientist (ICMR). He completed his Bachelor of Chemical Engineering (Hons.) and Master of Chemical Engineering (Gold Medalist) from Jadavpur University and went to Germany for carrying out his Doctoral Research as a DAAD Fellow, awarded Ph. D (Chemical Engineering) in 1982 and joined to the Pharmaceutical Technology Department, Jadavpur University as a Lecturer. Prof. Pal visited Darmstadt Technical University (Germany) as a DAAD Fellow (1978-81) under the invitation of German Academic Exchange Service and he had the opportunity to work with the eminent scientists Prof. (Dr.) Fritz Fetting in Germany as well as Dr. Endre Nagy, Dr. (Mrs.) Belafi K Bako, Dr. I. Salso and Dr. G. Laszlo of Hungary under the two Indo - Hungarian International projects (2000-03) & (2003-05) sponsored by DST, New Delhi. Dr. Pal also visited Germany and other European countries several times in connection with his Post-Doctoral research and presentation in the seminars / Conferences.

Prof. Pal had been doing research in the field of controlled release drug delivery Systems, pharmacokinetics, and bioequivalence studies since last 30 years with the financial support of Govt. funding agencies like DST, ICMR, UGC, and AICTE etc and got almost 7 Crore funds.

As a result of his continued research Prof. Pal has been able to publish more than 170 research papers in various National & International Journals and 51 students have been awarded Ph. D Degree under his supervision.

He founded the Bioequivalence Study Centre, Jadavpur University, the then only BA/BE Study Centre in eastern India approved by the CDSCO, Govt. of India. The analytical laboratory set up by Prof. Pal is equipped with all the sophisticated instruments like LC-MS/MS, HPLC, UV Spectrophotometer, Dissolution apparatus and other minor instruments and accessories required for Biopharmaceutical evaluation of drugs. Based on its excellent performance, the DCGI (Drugs Controller General of India) New Delhi has approved the laboratory for Bioequivalence studies in 2002. This laboratory had been carrying out B.E study on human volunteers by rendering services to more than 60 Pharmaceutical industries all over India as well as outside of India.

After his retirement he is now attached to this centre as Advisor cum Mentor. Three patents had been granted to him. He also wrote 3 books previously.

An eminent professor with great enthusiasm and energy even at the age of 70 is still very much active and still contributing to the pharmaceutical field by means of the technology and skilled manpower development (research scholars fit for the industry) under the purview of BA/BE study of generic drugs.

www.ingramcontent.com/pod-product-compliance
Lightning Source LLC
LaVergne TN
LVHW021704160726
843514LV00001B/249